Curanderismo

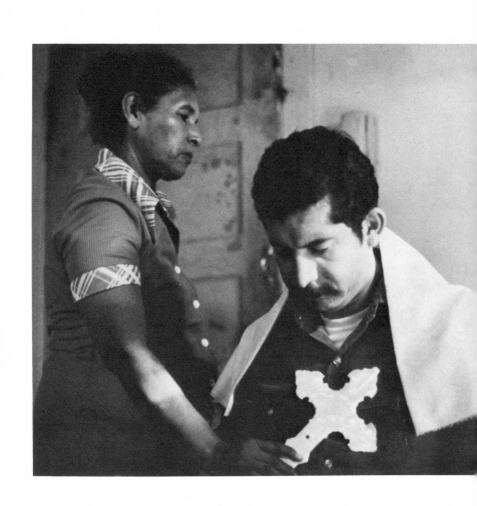

Robert T. Trotter II
and Juan Antonio Chavira

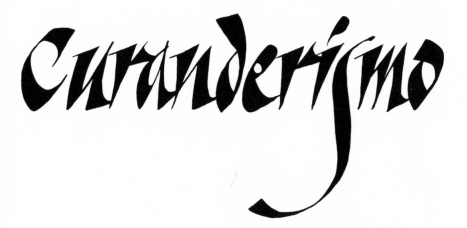

MEXICAN
AMERICAN
FOLK
HEALING

The University of Georgia Press
Athens

Copyright © 1981 by the University of Georgia Press
Athens, Georgia 30602

All rights reserved

Set in Trump Medieval type
Designed by Sandra Strother
Printed in the United States of America

Library of Congress Cataloging in Publication Data

Trotter, Robert T.
  Curanderismo, Mexican American folk healing.

  Includes index.
  1. Mexican American folk medicine.   2. Healing
(in religion, folk-lore, etc.)—United States.
I. Chavira, Juan Antonio.   II. Title.
GRI11.M49T76   398'.353   81-602
ISBN 0-8203-0556-1   AACR2
ISBN 0-8203-0570-7 (pbk.)

To the people of the Lower Rio Grande Valley of Texas

CONTENTS

ILLUSTRATIONS

PREFACE

THE DATA that support the information contained in this book, along with an associated film (*Los Que Curan*) and slide series (*Curanderismo: An Optional Health Care System*), were initially collected as a part of *Proyecto Comprender* (Regional Medical Program of Texas Grant 75-108G). A considerable amount of additional information has been collected in the four years since *Proyecto Comprender*.

Proyecto Comprender was developed to document the practices of Mexican American folk healers and to present this information as an educational package consisting of a film, a slide series, and a monograph on the Mexican American folk health-care system, *curanderismo*. The primary goal of the project was to lessen cultural barriers to the delivery of health care to Mexican American patients by providing health-care professionals and others with information that may help them understand events occurring in the lives of some of their patients. Within a short time after the beginning of the project, we discovered that only a small part of the total Mexican American system of folk medicine had been studied in depth, while other areas were either poorly represented in the literature or completely undocumented. This discovery changed the scope of the project dramatically. Unfortunately, we had only a limited amount of time to complete this project. Consequently, a number of areas within the *curanderismo* system were identified by the project which have not yet been fully researched. Other practices reported by informants during the research are not discussed here because we lacked rigorous, firsthand data pertaining to them. Far more research needs to be done on *curanderismo* before the complete relationship among beliefs, values, and health for Mexican Americans has been adequately documented and illustrated. Therefore, the information in this book should not be considered absolutely complete or immutable but merely a base or a starting point for further research.

The cooperation and hard work of a large number of people made this work possible, and we feel those people should be given the recognition they deserve. The Pan American University staff of *Proyecto Comprender* consisted of: Julian Castillo, director of the Division of Health Related Professions; Robert T. Trotter, II, project coordinator and coprincipal investigator, medical anthropologist; Juan Antonio Chavira, coprincipal investigator, medical sociologist-anthropologist; Aida Hurtado, research assistant and photographer; Liz R. Chavira, script writer for the slide series; Lucia Rodriguez, research assistant; Silverio Arenas, research assistant; Antonio Rivera, photographer; Esperanza Cantu, project secretary; and Olga O. Ambriz, division secretary. This manuscript has gone through several revisions, and we would like to thank Velma García and José Luiz González, our student assistants and secretaries, who helped tremendously by their speedy and accurate revisions of the manuscripts.

Others who contributed to the book through their expertise and knowledge of *curanderismo* include Jose Alfonso Treviño, Maria de la Luz-Rosalez, Maria Marta Balderas, Socorro Bravo, Jose Meave, Guadalupe Meave, Herminia Chavez-Blanco, Juventina Martínez, and many others. We would like to thank them for their help. They not only provided us with much detailed information, but also had the patience to allow us to repeat it to them and check for accuracy numerous times. The accurate details in the book are to their credit, while any mistakes are due to our inability to present what we have learned from them in an adequate fashion.

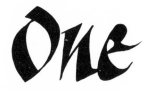

CURANDERISMO:
PAST AND PRESENT
VIEWPOINTS

CURANDERISMO, the Mexican American folk-healing system, is an important source of health resources for Mexican
Americans living in the Lower Rio Grande Valley of Texas
and other places. The term *curanderismo* and the term *curandero* come from the Spanish verb *curar*, which means
"to heal." Loosely, the word *curandero* could be applied to
anyone who claims to have some skill in the healing arts,
from a brain surgeon to a grandmother giving medicinal teas.
However, for Mexican Americans the title *curandero* represents a healer who is part of a historically and culturally important system of health care. Therefore, in this book the
word *curandero* is reserved for a person whose main profession and full-time work is as a healer, who sees more than
five patients a day, and who uses all or some significant part
of the theoretical system described here. The book itself is
an ethnography of the healing theories and practices of *curanderos* practicing in Mexican American communities in the
United States.

Curanderos have long been a community health resource
because the evolution and practice of *curanderismo* parallel
the historical and cultural evolution of Mexican Americans
as a population. The *curandero* is often a person chosen
from the community, who shares the same experiences, the

same language, and the same socioeconomic status as his or her patients. The *curandero* is highly accessible, without the intervening variables of excessive social and spatial distance that sometimes affect the delivery of health care in the United States. Usually, the only major distinctions between the *curandero* and the patient are the *curandero*'s healing powers and medicinal knowledge. The *curandero*'s office is in the community, normally in the healer's home. No appointments are necessary, referrals are not often required, no bureaucratic forms must be filled out, and no fees for services are charged (the patient gives a donation, using his conscience as his guide). The patient does not need to be covered by Medicare, Medicaid, Blue Cross, or the Kaiser plan to have access to the *curandero*.

Another characteristic that makes the *curandero* an important community health resource is the way that the healers use culturally appropriate methods of dealing with the patients, methods that activate the natural support system already existing in the community, rather than attempting to develop new or artificial support systems. The religious and spiritual aspects of the healing process capitalize on the patients' faith and belief systems. The use of herbs, fruits, eggs, and oils allows healing to occur through the use of everyday resources, products the patient can easily obtain. And by making themselves an integral part of the patient's existing social network, the *curanderos* can use the patient's family and peer group to support or implement the designated therapy.

The *curanderos'* practices and theories have evolved through centuries of services to patients in the community, often when the healer provided the only health care available. Within the past twenty years, at least in the Lower Rio Grande Valley, the socioeconomic position of many Mexican Americans has improved so that modern medical resources are increasingly available; widely utilized, and appreciated by both *curanderos* and patients, since modern medicine offers excellent care for a number of medical problems. However, at least in the valley, this use of modern medical facilities by both *curanderos* and their patients has not had the effect expected by some social scientists. *Curanderismo* has not disappeared. It continues to exist, thrive, and even evolve creative new forms of dealing with health and misfortune, side by side with modern medicine, and in (often silent) partnership with it.

In many respects the research supporting this book can be considered an urban ethnography, since it was conducted in the context of an urban-industrial system. The research area is the Lower Rio Grande Valley of Texas, near the mouth of the Rio Grande River. This is the flood plain of the Rio Grande River, and despite its name is totally devoid of even mild folds of land, let alone hills or mountains. On the United States side of the border, where the majority of the research was conducted, the valley is composed of three counties: Hidalgo, Cameron, and Willacy. Starr County is sometimes included in the valley area, but so little research was conducted in that area that it has been omitted for the purposes of this ethnography.

The valley has a somewhat unusual settlement pattern. A habitation strip no more than fifteen miles wide has been formed along the river by a nearly continuous series of small towns (populations ranging from 2,000 to 75,000) running from Brownsville at the mouth of the Rio Grande to Mission, approximately sixty-five miles upstream. This strip is bordered by, and often liberally interspersed with, citrus groves and agricultural fields, so the entire region is an inextricable rural-urban mixture. While agriculture remains the major industry of the area, using the extensive irrigation system made possible by the Rio Grande, the major urban centers of Brownsville and McAllen are important marketing, educational, and trade centers for south Texas and northern Mexico. The approximately half a million people in the area (79.1 percent Mexican American) live in a basically urban environment. The valley, however, maintains a strong rural quality: an estimated 80,000 migrant farm workers live there, and the area is also dotted with over a hundred rural, unincorporated villages called *colonias*. These *colonias* often lack potable water, proper drainage, sewage, and other modern utilities, as did other parts of the rural United States before rural electrification.

The Mexican side of the valley includes the northern region of the state of Tamaulipas. The pattern of settlement on the Mexican side is more clearly divided between rural and urban areas. The two large population centers of Matamoros (opposite Brownsville) and Reynosa (seven miles from McAllen) are important tourist, commercial, trade, and refining centers for northern Mexico. Matamoros is also a port city and the port of entry for oil and gas coming from Mexico to the United States. The area between Matamoros and Reynosa is largely rural, concentrating on grain and ranching. Rio Bravo, a city of about 50,000 between the two major cities, serves as the center of agricultural activity for this region.

Historically, the area has been a focus of cooperation and conflict between Mexico and the United States. Shifts of population back and forth are commonplace; tourists to Mexico, shoppers to the U.S., in the old days rustlers, smugglers, adventurers, and, always, people searching for a better life. Whatever the circumstances, the interaction of the two cultures has produced a unique bilingual-bicultural area; it is often hard to tell where one culture ends and the other begins. In this social environment old traditions die slowly, even as new ones are constantly introduced. In essence this area gives its residents a choice of languages, food, music, ways of life, and systems of healing that is paralleled by few other geographical populations in the United States.

In 1974 and 1975 the authors formed a research team with several student assistants to describe the existing practices of Mexican American folk healers in the Lower Rio Grande

Valley of Texas. The project was funded by the Regional Medical Program of Texas and was called *Proyecto Comprender*. *Proyecto Comprender* was designed to provide health-care professionals with easily accessible documentary evidence of the current practices of *curanderos*. Eventually our research went far beyond the project's original goals; however, the basis for all of the subsequent research was laid with *Proyecto Comprender* and the elements of the research program begun there deserve to be documented in some detail.

The primary goal of *Proyecto Comprender* was to weaken cultural barriers to the delivery of health care to Mexican American patients by providing health-care professionals and others with information regarding the beliefs and practices of some of their patients. We assumed that these beliefs and practices, represented in the folk-healing system, had a direct effect on what patients expected of the health professional and of modern medical services. We also assumed that the professional might not be aware of these expectations through lack of contact with this traditional system. Of special interest were the theories, beliefs, values, symbols, and other forms of communication used by *curanderos*. We expected that this new knowledge would be useful to health professionals in their treatment of some of their Mexican American patients.

Before beginning the project we were certain that extensive research had been done on Mexican American folk medicine, but that the findings of such research were inaccessible to most health professionals, since such findings are usually buried in academic journals or available only through personal contact with the researchers involved in various studies. Therefore, the original goal of *Proyecto Comprender* was simply to redocument the available information and make it more accessible. That goal changed drastically when we discovered that major areas of *curanderismo* remained undocumented. And those previously undocumented areas of *curanderismo* suggested a broader base of participation in this system of folk medicine than was formerly assumed. Therefore the project expanded to include researching and documenting these unexplored areas, re-documenting the better-researched areas, and providing the broadest possible base of information to accomplish the original goals of the research.

The early research approach to *curanderos* had another, less expected shortcoming. Most of the research staff were Mexican Americans, confident of their knowledge and experiences with *curanderos*. However, Mexican Americans, like members of all other cultural groups, participate intensively in segmented aspects of their culture. As far as folk medicine is concerned, most of the researchers remember the *barridas*, the *yerbitas*, the *emplastes* they experienced in their youth without fully realizing what was happening or why. They accepted many aspects of their culture on faith and thereby became only superficially acquainted with specific things such as *curanderismo*. Previous experiences, therefore, did not prepare us for what we were to find in the field.

The purpose of collecting these data was neither to justify *curanderismo* nor to destroy it. It was simply to document it from a perspective as close to that of the healers as possible. Far more research needs to be done in the area of the relationship between specific medical conditions and the therapeutic techniques of the *curanderos* before the efficacy of folk healing is demonstrated. From that perspective, this study should be seen as a starting point for further research, a framework for organizing future studies.

Looking back, we can attribute the fact that *curanderismo* was not as well researched as expected, despite an extensive literature, to the underlying methodological approach that was taken by earlier researchers. It is clear from reading the available texts that *curanderismo* has been viewed and analyzed primarily as a mass-cultural phenomenon, not as a coherent system. It has been treated as a body of knowledge that is widely distributed throughout the Mexican American culture and, like cooking or courting, is available to and used by a significant segment of the population. This view of folk medicine tends to make any discussion of the topic nontheoretical, at least in terms of expecting or eliciting an emic theory of *curanderismo*, because while systems (for example, medical, educational, and scientific systems) are easily recognized as depending on theory, mass-cultural phenomena are generally thought of as having themes or unifying elements, but not theories. Mass-cultural phenomena are something one has theories about, but they are not theoretical systems themselves.

This viewpoint is well represented in the articles about *curanderismo* that reflect its form or function within Mexican American communities (for example, Clark 1959, 1959b; Currier 1966; Edgerton et al. 1970; Foster 1953; Kiev 1968; Madsen 1961, 1964; Martinez and Martin 1966; Rubel 1960, 1964, 1966; Romano 1965; and Torrey 1969). Because of the mass-cultural approach, the vast majority of these authors (and those in the appended bibliography) provide a highly repetitious and shallow perspective of *curanderismo*, overemphasizing the well-known (by now) Mexican American "cultural illnesses": *susto, empacho, mal de ojo, caida de mollera, bilis,* and *espanto* (see Nall 1967:302 for definitions).

The overemphasizing of these folk illnesses in the literature is probably due to their accessibility. None of these diseases is controversial or socially threatening; they form an easy topic of conversation. In fact, talking about these folk illnesses can be used to steer the conversation away from more sensitive topics. In addition, many of the activities connected with these illnesses, such as touching a baby after admiring it to prevent *mal ojo,* are highly visible and would naturally attract the attention of a trained observer. Thus, one gets the impression that some anthropologists were figuratively made to sit in a corner and given enough interesting, but nonthreatening, information to keep them from digging hard enough to uncover more sensitive or controversial issues in the community.

Little effort seems to have been made by previous authors to go beyond a description of the folk illnesses to demonstrate the links between recognizing the presence of disease, diagnosing it, identifying its cause, and treating it. This situation is analogous to doing anthropological research on surgery by focusing on the perceptions of the patient only. Such a project would produce valid descriptions of a mass cultural phenomenon, but would probably miss the theoretical elements of medicine that would be better learned from the specialist performing the surgery. Such an analysis would tend to emphasize disparate elements of surgery that did not appear bound by a common theme, just as *mal de ojo, empacho, susto,* and so forth have been presented as disparate entities, lacking a coherent binding theory.

In contrast, we directed our research almost entirely at the *curanderos.* Having assumed that *curanderismo,* like medicine, exists because people are ill and want help, we aimed our research at the *curanderos'* definitions of illness, their concepts of health and bodily functions, their procedures for treatment, their beliefs, and their training processes. From the beginning our objectives for gathering data were fourfold:

1. to identify the majority of known and respected local *curanderos,* who were defined as professionals
2. to interview representatives of the major specializations within *curanderismo,* in depth
3. to observe healing interactions extensively as participants
4. to do in-depth case studies of a few *curanderos.*

The professional *curanderos* were identified by their reputations and by lay referrals. In identifying known and respected *curanderos* two community sources of information became important. First, we consulted our own friends and acquaintances in the *barrios* of different cities in the Lower Rio Grande Valley; second, we consulted the relatives, friends, and acquaintances of our students at Pan American University. Thus we obtained lists of names and addresses of people considered to be good, reliable *curanderos*.

Since the research has been going on for over six years, this technique of identifying healers has been extremely successful. More than sixty healers have been interviewed. These healers include *parteras* (midwives), *yerberos* (herbalists), *sobadores* (people who treat sprains and strained muscles), and the group defined as *curanderos*, who manipulate the supernatural world as well as the physical world.

Whenever we were asked why we wanted to talk to *curanderos*, we gave these reasons:

1. We wanted to document and preserve an important characteristic of Mexican American culture.
2. We were working on a project that would disseminate information to public health and medical personnel, so that they would be better able to understand Mexican American concepts of health and illness, and perhaps be better able to provide services for Mexican Americans.
3. We wanted to learn as much (both professionally and personally) as the *curandero* would teach us.
4. We wanted to know what the *curandero* considered to be important as far as health and illness were concerned.
5. We wanted to know the level of need that exists for the *curandero's* services.
6. We wanted to know why people seek the services of a *curandero*.

In most instances a *curandero* was interviewed only after an intermediary first asked for his or her consent. In a few instances the *curanderos* refused to be interviewed. The most common reasons for refusal were fear of being reported to the medical establishment, fear of being ridiculed, and lack of time to talk to the researchers. At no time did any member of the research team feign illness, nor did anyone invent a problem to gain access to a *curandero*. At no time did we intend to mislead anyone about the purpose of the study or about the way we meant to use the information gathered.

The data contained in this paper were elicited through participant observation combined with key informant interviewing to uncover the logical premises of *curanderismo*. Two important individuals provided the initial structuring of the theoretical orientation presented here. These individuals were chosen as key informants because of their willingness to work with the authors on a long-term basis and because of their apparent success as healers. Both enjoy good reputations in their community, and both had been healing for more than ten years when they were initially contacted. One is male, the other female. The male lives in Reynosa but travels at least one day a week to a town in the United States to consult with patients there. The female lived in Edinburg while the project was in progress, only a few blocks from Pan American University; afterwards she moved to another town close by. Each sees from ten to fifty patients a day, and, as far as we could tell, they had not had any contacts with one another prior to and during much of the research project. All of the data collected from these and other informants were and still are being cross-checked and verified constantly.

Throughout the initial interviews we ourselves were encouraged to learn the healing process. The entire research team was given a series of tests, by nearly every *curandero* interviewed, to see if any had the gift of healing. One test involved our sitting in a semicircle with palms open upward, resting on our laps, and with our eyes closed. The *curandero* stood in front of the group, a clear glass filled with water nearby, and said invocations to the spiritual realm. Each member of the group was told to concentrate on the

Supreme Being and to remain sitting in this fashion for about fifteen minutes. At the end of this session each one was asked to describe the sensations he or she felt. The *curandero* thought that one of the members of the research group had the potential to be a medium because of that person's sensations, actions, and certain vibrations perceived only by the *curandero*. Through this experience and others like it, several members of the research staff were offered the opportunity to learn healing techniques with the different realms of *curanderismo*. In fact, both of the authors were invited to act as apprentices to one or the other of the two key informants. This opportunity may have been largely responsible for our discovering the theory of *curanderismo*, since an apprentice must not only learn what he has to do, he is also expected to learn why he does it, and, especially, why it is done one particular way and not another.

The first part of the research was intensive interviewing. The informants were soon aware of our ignorance and dependence on misleading information about *curanderismo* and misdirections for research questions from the previous literature. But they were both patient. Initially, the healers often appeared to ignore the point of many of the questions and to give vague or general answers. It was a somewhat frustrating experience, but eventually a pattern of information became apparent and it turned out that the healers had been presenting a coherent body of information, starting with general concepts and terminology and gradually moving to specific details once the general information was assimilated.

A second consideration slowed our attempts to probe into *curanderismo* during this first phase. One *curandero* said it very well: "Many of these things you must experience, before you understand them. When you have experienced and understood them, you either will not need to ask questions, or your questions will be the kind that I can answer." These initial interviews were unstructured and open-ended, addressing themselves to specific topics using whatever questions seemed necessary at the time. All interviews were recorded and then transcribed. Examples of these interviews include a taped, four-hour conversation on the use of herbs, a three-hour conversation on the use of candles, a spiritual session lasting two and a half hours, and two hours on how to protect houses, businesses, and livestock. In this phase of the research more than sixty-five hours of taped information were collected, constituting in-depth studies of the knowledge, concepts, theories, and tools that the *curanderos* use in treating their patients, not to mention notes from untaped interviews. Several thousand feet of movie film depicting curing procedures, as well as over 2,500 still photographs, were also collected. This initial collection of data has been augmented by continued interviews and research on specific problems during the four years since *Proyecto Comprender* was completed.

The second step in our observation of *curanderismo* began with a series of nine *limpias* or spiritual cleansings. These *limpias* were to prepare us to receive spiritual communication and cleanse our bodies from harm or evil. Then began the observation of healing rituals, participation in spiritual sessions, and the learning of actual prayers, rituals, and diagnostic interpretations used in treatment. Many of these healing rituals and procedures were recorded during actual healing sessions.

Photographic documentation at all these sessions was possible, but problematic. The general anthropological literature on healing led us to expect that entry into the healing system would be difficult and that informants would probably not tolerate tape recordings and certainly not photographs or films and videotapes to be taken. Our experience was just the opposite. We got a surprisingly warm welcome because, as one informant told us, the *curanderos* had a number of things that they wanted the medical establishment to know. We were encouraged to record sessions and admonished not to forget our tape recorders for future sessions. Photographs were permitted far more frequently than we had expected, although some patients who would let us observe did not want to be photographed.

Films and videotape presented the most serious problems, but the difficulties there were caused not by extraordinary reluctance on the part of the *curanderos*, but by the physical characteristics of the equipment and the need for rather uncomfortable light levels when filming indoors, where most of the healing takes place. In some cases it was possible to photograph actual *curandero*-patient interaction; in other cases it was necessary to simulate healing conditions: the *curandero* executed the rituals and procedures exactly as he would have in an actual cure but this time for the sole purpose of being filmed or photographed. Sometimes actual patients were filmed; at other times the role of the patient was taken by one of the researchers. It was impossible to document certain ritual settings because of their sensitivity and the intrusiveness of a flash unit or the noise of motion-picture photography. Under these circumstances we made no attempt to impose on the healers by demanding the impossible or the impolite. In addition to some of the technical and procedural problems encountered in documenting our research, the simple fact is that the reality of *curanderismo* is sometimes difficult to photograph. The spiritual and mental levels are especially difficult. Whenever these highly abstract and invisible levels were reached, the subjective reports of our informants became more important than our own observations—a situation that makes social scientists uncomfortable, at best, but a situation that is common to most ethnographies of folk medicine.

Certain data from previous studies were confirmed by the authors. These data include the existence and treatment of the so-called folk illnesses of Mexican Americans (*empacho*, *susto*, and so forth; see Nall 1967); however, we found these illnesses to be of relatively minor importance in the healing system. The individuals we define as *curanderos* seldom treat these diseases because, as one informant put it, "anyone can take care of those things. We only see the ones that other people, the mother, the grandmothers, the neighbor, cannot cure." Instead, the *curanderos* are sought out to deal with problems of a much more serious nature.

The study also corroborated the information that the healers' perspective of health and illness contains a dual element of "natural" and "supernatural" illnesses. This duality forms the base upon which *curanderismo* is structured. "The members of *La Raza* [Mexican Americans] do not divide the natural and the supernatural into separate compartments as Anglos do. A harmonious relationship between the natural and the supernatural is considered essential to human health and welfare, while disharmony precipitates illness and misfortune" (Madsen 1964:68).

The *curanderos'* concept of the natural source of illness overlaps extensively with the medical model. Such basic premises of modern medicine as the germ theory of disease are accepted. Natural illnesses are seen as being amenable to treatment by physicians, by herbal remedies, and occasionally through supernatural intervention, although the last is not the preferred mode since it takes time and energy that could be better spent on other cures.

The *curanderos* do not consider supernatural sources of illness amenable to treatment by the medical establishment. The *curanderos* indicated that any particular illness suffered by a patient could theoretically be caused by either natural or supernatural processes. This means that there is a natural form of diabetes and a form caused by a supernatural agent, such as a *brujo* (witch or sorcerer). The same is true for alcoholism, cancer, and so on. One of the key problems that the *curanderos* deal with is identifying the nature of the causal agent for a particular illness.

The *curanderos* recognize that their acceptance of magic and witchcraft makes them an object of ridicule from the

scientific medical system. They feel this ridicule is not jus-
tified, and they fault the medical system for its lack of attention to the supernatural. One *curandero* went so far as to say
that many of the people in mental institutions (he estimated
10 percent) were there because they were *embrujados*
(hexed persons), but the doctors could not recognize this
condition, so it went untreated. Supernaturally caused illnesses were most commonly said to be initiated by either
evil spirits (*espiritus malos*) or by *brujos,* and these provoked illnesses form a significant part of the *curanderos'*
work on the United States side of the border.

Some *curanderos* appear to identify more supernatural
causes for illnesses than others do. A student once asked
one of us to take him to a key informant. The student very
strongly felt he was *embrujado* (hexed) by a former girl
friend whom he had treated poorly. The student was in poor
health; he was failing his courses; he was always tired. He
presented these symptoms to the *curandero* and asked that
the *trabajo* (magical work or hex) be removed. The *curandero* examined the student using his magical training
and then asked him a series of questions about his habits:
whether he went to many parties, how much he drank, how
much he studied. The *curandero* very bluntly told the student that he could find absolutely no supernatural cause for
his troubles. He said that the student's problems were directly the effect of too many parties, too much drinking, not
enough studying, and lack of sleep. If he concentrated on
work and study, the student's condition would improve
enormously.

This also illustrates that the authors were able to confirm
Holland's (1963) and Kiev's (1968) reports that there is far
less dichotomizing of physical and social problems within
curanderismo than within the medical-care system. The
curanderos very clearly deal with social, psychological, and
spiritual problems as well as with physical ailments. In
many cases the problems overlap into two or more catego-

ries. Bad luck in business was a common problem presented to the *curanderos*. They also had to deal with marital disruptions, alcoholism, infidelity, bothersome supernatural manifestations, cancer, diabetes, and infertility. The list of problems presented to the *curanderos* is nearly inexhaustible. Obviously, Galvin (1961), Kline (1969), Torrey (1972) and many others are correct in saying that *curanderismo* plays an important, culturally appropriate psychotherapeutic role in some Mexican American communities.

Another previously described element of *curanderismo* that was supported by the present study is the belief in the existence of "a gift of healing" (*el don*) that provides the *curandero* with his or her ability to heal. This concept was reported by Hudson (1951) and Romano (1964) for an extremely important and famous south Texas folk healer, Don Pedrito Jaramillo (1829–1907). It is also reported in a more general way by Madsen (1964a), Rubel (1966), and others. The *don* is the basic difference between the healer and nonhealer; it allows the healer to practice his or her work, especially in the supernatural area. It is clear that the *don* for healing in the past was felt to be a gift from God. However, a secular interpretation of the presence of the *don* is now competing with the more traditional explanation. Many healers still refer to the *don* as a gift from God and support this premise by reference to biblical passages (for example, 1 Corinthians 12:7 and James 5:14). Other healers explain the *don* as an inborn trait that is common to and present in all human beings. They consider it to have the same basis as singing, running, or talking. Almost any human being can do these activities, but some obviously can do them better than others, and a few can do them extremely well. *Curanderos*, according to these healers, are simply the individuals with a better ability to heal than is normative for the population as a whole. The healers refer to this condition as having "developed abilities."

One element of Hispanic folk medicine that is present in

most areas, the hot-cold syndrome (see Ingham 1940; Foster 1953; and Currier 1966), is missing in south Texas. This unexpected finding was first noted by Madsen (1961:23–24) and was corroborated by our own data. No healers who were raised in the area made use of the hot-cold dichotomy to explain illness, although it was used in organizing herbal cures by one informant who was born in central Mexico and migrated to the valley as an adult. The only elements of the hot-cold syndrome that the authors found were a few scattered beliefs about women not eating citrus when having their period, or not taking a cold shower after being in the hot sun. No systematic use of the hot-cold concepts were otherwise documented.

Since most of this work is devoted to an ethnographic description of *curanderismo* from the viewpoint of the healers, it seems worthwhile to also provide information on how *curanderismo* is viewed from the perspectives of nonhealers. Thus we shall begin by exposing at least some of the social environment and expressing some of the attitudes that surround *curanderismo* in the valley. We found that by the very nature of its unofficial and unsanctioned status in relation to conventional modern healing systems, it tends to be a controversial subject. It is a subject that can elicit strong responses, both positive and negative, based on the perspective of the individual evaluating the subject. The evaluator's perspective in turn depends on the specific role or function he or she believes *curanderismo* performs, as well as on his or her previous experiences with it.

Curanderos, like all health-care professionals, are perceived from at least three viewpoints. One viewpoint is that of the general nonparticipating public. In a multicultural or a multiethnic environment, this viewpoint depends on whether the viewer has a cultural background similar to or different from the system of folk medicine being studied. In either case this viewpoint can be called the outsider's perspective. The second viewpoint is the perspective of those who are participant-patients of the *curanderos*. This can be called the client's perspective. The third viewpoint on *curanderismo* is the perspective of the *curanderos* themselves. This is the practitioner's perspective.

The most varied perspective on *curanderismo* is the view from the outside. For people with different cultural experiences, this view is often based on myth, superstition, and social stereotypes. In many cases there is a complete lack of information about *curanderismo* even among Anglo-Americans who have spent their entire lives in south Texas. In other cases the picture is distorted through a cultural filter and through incomplete experience or knowledge of the system. This is not unexpected, since this is the common condition for cross-cultural understanding in multiethnic environments, especially when one culture defines itself as superior to the other.

It would be nearly impossible to document all of the views which the general public holds regarding *curanderos*. For our purposes we have divided outsiders into three categories: the critics, the doubters, and the pragmatists. However, we will discuss only what may be considered the most salient features of each category, since most of these viewpoints tend to blend into each other.

The most outspoken and hostile critics of *curanderismo* are usually those who do not believe in the *curandero's* practices. The reasons for their skepticism vary: denial of the reality of what *curanderismo* is and what the *curanderos* do, disbelief in the moral validity of the system, rejection on the basis of sociocultural stereotypes of Mexican Americans, and concern over the effect of *curanderismo* on patients in need of medical care.

Those who reject *curanderos* on the basis of social stereotypes consider them purveyors of ignorance and superstition and major contributors to the existence of a culture that should have been discarded long ago. This rejection indicates a strong tendency toward assimilation. In essence,

Mexican American culture is viewed by these people as being inferior; they tend to reject anything and anyone who continues to keep it alive. Therefore they reject *curanderismo* because it reinforces and justifies the existence of what is thought to be ignorant superstition and mumbo-jumbo nonsense. Many of these people appear to accept modern medicine not because it is thought to be a better or a more efficient system, but because it is a symbol of entrance into a superior culture.

Other people reject *curanderismo* because they believe *curanderos* to be frauds and quacks. Some believe all *curanderos* are frauds, preying on the gullibility of people and taking away their money by promising wondrous results. These people are often concerned that the *curandero's* clients may lose money to an unscrupulous healer whose only purpose is to make a quick buck. Others, viewing all *curanderos* as quacks, are concerned for the client's health. These people suggest that the sick lose time, money, and sometimes their lives by going to someone who really cannot help them. They are also concerned that people may be taking medication prescribed by the *curanderos*, which may be ineffective in relieving pain or may have harmful effects when used with drugs prescribed by a physician. Thus all *curanderos* are labeled as frauds, as quacks, because they are thought to harm rather than to help people.

Some people reject *curanderos* because of the mystery surrounding the source of their power; many consider them agents of the devil. Their healing powers, their magical powers, their source of knowledge, are all believed to be part of a cult or a false religion and in direct opposition to the tenets of various churches, especially the fundamentalist sects. The fundamentalists often view participating in *curanderismo* as analogous to worshipping idols and strange gods. In this case, the rejector feels that the best thing to do is to keep away from *curanderos*, since they are inspired by the devil as a trap for unwary believers.

Some people are ambivalent toward *curanderismo*: those who are afraid someone may laugh at them for believing in a marginal superstition and those who are honestly not sure of *curanderismo*'s value. Both of these groups tend to view the practices with some degree of skepticism but do not reject them outright. Examples of the acculturated doubter can be found in the ranks of Mexican American college students who come from very traditional *barrio* environments and who as children were at least partially initiated into this healing system. As adolescents they tend to leave their *barrio* culture seeking a new identity in a more acculturated school atmosphere. They generally admit the existence of *curanderismo* and probably have relatives and family members who are very much a part of the system. However, they are afraid to admit they have participated for fear of being ridiculed by others. Nonetheless, the family socialization process keeps their doubts from turning into utter disbelief despite their relatively high level of education. This type of doubting sometimes occurs among professionals and other working adults.

Some doubters have actually seen *curanderos* perform successful cures, but they remain unconvinced of the value of *curanderismo*. They may be afraid of getting involved or afraid to openly admit that *curanderismo* works in some cases. A great number have witnessed the successful cure of *mal ojo*, while others have seen more spectacular cures of people who could not walk or could not move.

Some people appreciate the therapeutic value of *curanderismo* but do not believe that the *curandero* has any power of his own. They believe the *curandero*'s power comes from the people's faith in him. These doubters usually say they would never go to a *curandero* but would not criticize or interfere with those who seek a *curandero*'s help. They believe the *curandero* is really not helping directly; the people are helping themselves through the power of their own minds. Thus, the value of the *curandero* is as a psychosomatic healer.

There are many people in the community who are skeptical about *curanderismo* but want to know more about it. These skeptics can be divided into two groups: the scientifically oriented and the spiritually oriented. The scientific skeptic is not sure if *curanderismo* works, but would like to empirically assess the *curandero's* theories and his therapeutic techniques. The spiritually oriented skeptic is interested in the *curandero's* premise that spiritual harmony is essential to good health, yet the source of the *curandero's* power to some degree either frightens him or makes him wary of pursuing his interest.

To greater or lesser degree all these people find themselves stranded between two orientations: the scientific-rational reality of our educational system, which tends to discount the reality of *curanderismo*, and the humanistic, faith-oriented reality of their early socialization period, which tends to reinforce the reality of *curanderismo*.

The third group we call the pragmatists, whose identifying characteristic is that they have the welfare of the sick as their primary goal. Their major concern is to include in the health-care system anything that will make the treatment of patients more effective. Some of these people believe that *curanderos* can help in the treatment of the sick and should therefore be incorporated into the medical system. Others want to find out first whether the *curanderos* really can provide therapeutic relief to the patients. If they can help either in actual treatment or in convincing people to seek treatment, then perhaps a system of cooperation should be established. If the *curanderos* do no harm they can be tolerated; if they harm rather than heal, then the necessary steps should be taken to prevent their being used as a health resource.

Several views of *curanderismo* are held by those who are either active or passive participants in the system.

These views differ because not everyone goes to *curanderos* with the same expectations, nor are all treatments equally successful.

Some people participate in *curanderismo* because they are taken to the healers by friends and relatives who believe in the system. Others go merely to satisfy their own curiosity about *curanderos*. Those who seek *curanderos* out of curiosity usually see neither harm nor benefit from their participation. Some even hover around the system, taking friends or relatives for help without actually seeking treatment for themselves. Other passive participants are those who have no control over their actions but are brought to the *curandero* by concerned relatives. These patients may be children, the elderly, the mentally retarded, or the mentally disturbed. These patients usually come from families who are strong believers or from families who go to the *curandero* as a last resort. Such people tend to have neutral attitudes toward *curanderismo* until their participation provides them with experiences that convince them about the good or the harm that *curanderismo* produces.

Many of the participants in the folk medical system are believers. Those who believe in *curanderismo* are often long-time users of the system. They seek *curanderos* because they believe in the *curandero*'s theories and definitions of illness and because they have faith in the therapeutic techniques of the *curandero*. Moreover, the believers usually testify that they have been helped by the *curanderos*. They continue to seek *curanderos* because they are satisfied patients. By performing successful and sometimes apparently miraculous cures, *curanderos* reinforce the believers' already positive attitudes toward the folk-healing system.

Curanderismo, like all professions, has its share of quacks and con artists who are experts at exploiting the faith and inexperience of their clients. Patients who are cheated often come to the healer with a rather serious problem, expecting some kind of miracle. Dishonest *curanderos*, knowing the vulnerability of persons seeking quick solutions for serious problems, promise more than they can deliver in order to make a quick profit. Their patients not only lose money, but also fail to achieve their expectations. As a result they become doubly cheated—emotionally and financially—and they are usually vehement in their condemnation of *curanderismo*.

Our review of the literature on *curanderismo* clearly showed that the viewpoints of the *curanderos* themselves had been seriously neglected by researchers. This is one of the conditions that this book aims to rectify. Most of our information was gathered directly from the *curanderos*. While there are many differences among *curanderos* on the origin, extent, and utilization of their abilities, we were able to identify some of their more common themes and perspectives.

Many *curanderos* think of themselves as agents doing the work of God. These *curanderos* claim that their healing powers are a gift from God and that all their success can be attributed to the mercy and power of the Lord. As a gift from God, their powers can be neither exploited nor used to harm anyone. These *curanderos* feel that they have a moral obligation to help those in need, to relieve the misery of those who are suffering, and to counsel those in distress.

In reality *curanderos* can only try to live up to this ideal. Many difficulties intrude on their behavior. Survival is expensive now, so they must often charge for their services, whereas there is some indication that in the past no charges were made at all. Moreover, most *curanderos* have families and dependents who need the basic necessities of life, not only food and shelter but also attention and love. The pressures of having people calling at all hours of the day, every day of the week, can sometimes become a nuisance. As one of our informants told us, "Sometimes I wish I were like everyone else." He added that the responsibility of having so many people dependent on him for so many things is often too great. It deprives him of time with his family, especially his children, and of time to pursue his other interests. There are patients who become so dependent on him that they will not leave him alone. There are times when he wants to do something else so badly that he does not dedicate as much time as he feels he should to his patients.

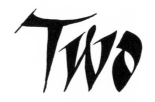

THE
HISTORY OF
CURANDERISMO

AT LEAST SIX MAJOR HISTORICAL INFLUENCES have shaped the beliefs and practices of *curanderismo* by Mexican Americans in the Lower Rio Grande Valley: Judeo-Christian religious beliefs, symbols, and rituals; early Arabic medicine and health practices (combined with Greek humoral medicine, revived during the Spanish Renaissance); medieval and later European witchcraft; Native American herbal lore and health practices; modern beliefs about spiritualism and psychic phenomena; and scientific medicine. None of these influences dominates *curanderismo*, but each has had some impact on its historical development.

Judeo-Christian beliefs and practices provide the basic framework for *curanderismo*, just as for most Western cultural systems. The Bible and the teachings of the Church have been combined with folk wisdom to produce a foundation for the theories of both illness and healing that make up much of the structure of *curanderismo*.

The Bible has greatly influenced *curanderismo* through references made to the specific healing properties of animal parts, plants, oil, and wine (for example, see Luke 10:34). Humans are clearly instructed to use the resources, beginning with the general principle set forth in Genesis 1:29–31 that all the plants and animals were created for man's use and reinforced with the specific statement, "The Lord has created medicines from the earth, and a sensible man will not disparage them" (Ecclus. 38 : 4).

The pharmacological information in the Bible is fairly extensive for that time, but it is less important in its influence on *curanderismo* than are the basic concepts of healing embodied in the Bible. The principal concept found there can be termed "God's power over man." There are two aspects to this concept: first, the belief that God can and does heal directly; and second, the idea that people with a special gift from God can heal in his name.

The first method, healing through divine intervention, is common in the Bible. It is often used as a sign of God's presence among the masses. Such signs include the examples of Jesus' healing found in the New Testament:

> Wherever he went, to farmsteads, villages, or towns, they laid out the sick in the market places and begged him to let them simply touch the edge of his cloak; and all who touched him were cured. [Mark 6 : 56]

The second biblical foundation for folk healing, the healing power of faith, originates in the Apostles' instructions to the Church after Jesus' death. In these instructions, healing was directly linked to faith in God and in prayer:

> Is one of you ill? He should send for the elders of the congregation to pray over him and anoint him with oil in the name of the Lord. The prayer offered in faith will save the sick man, the Lord will raise him from his bed, and any sins he may have committed will be forgiven. [James 5 : 14]

Similar passages provide the rationalization for the existence of Mexican American folk healers as individuals, not as a part of the organization of the Church itself. Several *curanderos* referred to the following passage in the Bible to justify and explain their activities:

In each of us the Spirit is manifested in one particular
way, for some useful purpose. One man, through the
Spirit, has the gift of wise speech, while another, by the
power of the same Spirit, can put the deepest knowledge
into words. Another, by the same Spirit, is granted faith;
another, by the one Spirit, gifts of healing, and another
miraculous powers; another has the gift of prophecy, and
another ability to distinguish true spirits from false; yet
another has the gift of ecstatic utterance of different
kinds, and another the ability to interpret it. But all
these gifts are the work of one and the same Spirit, dis-
tributing them separately to each individual at will.
[1 Cor. 12:7–11]

Today these biblical principles are found in the healing
beliefs and practices of many (but not all) modern *curanderos*. These healers explain that their healing abilities are a
gift (*don*) from God, and that they heal through his power
and through the patient's belief in God (see Hudson 1951 on
Don Pedrito Jaramillo).

The concept of the soul, which is central to the teachings
of Christianity, also contributes to the *curandero*'s theories
of healing, in particular those cures performed by *curanderos* working as spiritualists (*espiritistas* and *espiritualistas*). Belief in the soul affirms the existence of saints and
devils, as well as the immortal soul of ordinary human
beings. The belief that souls or spirits (*espiritos*) can either
aid or hinder the healer promotes the desire or need for *curanderos* to contact them and petition them to use their
powers for good or evil ends. While the idea of the soul has a
strong biblical base, it was greatly expanded during medieval
and modern times and has become a part of the shamanism
and sorcery found in modern *curanderismo*.

Finally, the constant biblical theme of the dual worlds of
light and darkness, good and evil, health and illness, life and
death runs throughout the practice of *curanderismo*. This
symbolic system links all of the areas of *curanderismo* to-

gether. To heal may be a sign from God, since health is linked to light and goodness. To harm someone is to work in the absence of light (*un trabajo obscuro o negro*). Such an act promotes evil and illness. This dichotomy between good and evil is expressed on each of the levels of power recognized by both the Bible and by *curanderismo*: on the human level the *curandero* heals and the *brujo* (witch or sorcerer) harms; on the spiritual level benevolent souls and saints can bring luck, health, and contentment, while malevolent souls and demons bring misfortune, illness, and misery; on the highest level of existence God (the light and giver of health) opposes Satan and his evil works. Within *curanderismo* this duality presents a constant theme of oppositions integral to understanding it.

Preconquest Spain had the best-regarded system of medicine available in the Western world. The Spanish healing system combined earlier Greek and Roman practices of Hippocratic medicine with the highly successful Arabic medical practices introduced in Spain by the Moors. The Spanish medical theories and practices were brought to the New World at the time of the conquest and were eventually influenced by Native American healing practices.

Anthropologist George Foster (1953) notes the major theoretical components of the Hippocratic base of Spanish medical beliefs.

> The Hippocratian doctrine of the four "humors"—blood, phlegm, black bile ("melancholy"), and yellow bile ("choler")—formed the basis of medical theory. Each humor had its "complexion": blood, hot and wet; phlegm, cold and wet; black bile, cold and dry; yellow bile, hot and dry. . . . Natural history classification was rooted in the concept that people and even illness, medications, foods, and most natural objects had complexions. Thus, medical practice consisted largely of understanding the natural complexion of the patient, in determining the complexion of the illness or its cause, and in restoring

the fundamental harmony which had been disturbed.
[Foster 1953:202–3]

During the introduction of these medical beliefs into the
New World, the duality of wet and dry was for all practical
purposes lost. The continuing importance of the hot-cold
syndrome has been emphasized repeatedly in the literature
about Latin American folk medical beliefs (see Ingham
1940; Foster 1953; Currier 1966). However, the importance
of the hot-cold dichotomies varies from area to area and is
especially weak in south Texas. Even though one can find in
Mexican American communities in south Texas residual
folk sayings and household beliefs that reflect this hot-cold
dichotomy, it does not play a central part in the theoretical structure of *curanderismo*. This absence is noted by
Madsen:

> Hippocratic medicine was introduced into Mexico in the
> 16th century and is still a basic part of Mexican folk
> medicine but is of little significance in Mexican Ameri-
> can folk medicine of South Texas. Minor stomach upsets
> are believed to be caused by eating too many hot or cold
> foods in most communities, but the hot-cold complex is
> completely lacking in some localities. [Madsen
> 1961:23–24]

Similar results were obtained from our own research, although a continuing emphasis was placed on both the hot-
cold (and even with one *curandera*, the wet-dry dichotomies)
by people knowledgeable about herbal remedies (*yerberos*).

The Hispano-Arabic medical system contributed two important theories to Mexican American folk medicine. First,
it contributed the idea that health consists of a balanced
condition. The lack of harmony with the environment (social and spiritual as well as physical) produces illness, and
the readjustment or removal of this imbalance becomes the
primary function of the healer. Thus the basic tenets of *curanderismo* are to produce and protect a holistic relation-

ship between the individual and his total environment. Second, Spanish medical theory contributed the idea that medicinal remedies can be discovered in plants and animals, an idea that is reinforced by the teachings of the Bible. This emphasis on herbal medicines caused many individuals to search out and experiment with new sources of medicine in both the Old World and the New. These two themes, the restoration of health through the restoration of balance to the patient and the experimentation with and use of herbal remedies, have had an enduring influence on the practice of *curanderismo*.

The major symbols used in the rituals of *curanderos* (numbers, words, and objects), the structure of those rituals, and the theoretical explanations given for success in healing substantiate the importance of Old World historical influences on Mexican American folk medicine. The symbols used in healing rituals are overwhelmingly part of the Western cultural tradition. The numbers most frequently used to designate the length of cures, number of times rituals are performed, and other magical sequences of activities are all within the Judeo-Christian system of symbolic numbers (primarily 3, 7, 9, and 11; occasionally 13 for certain negative magical rites). Many of the objects used to promote healing are of Old World origin: olive oil, lemons, garlic, chickens, camomile, votive candles, and the crucifix, to name a few. Finally, the structure and theory of the *curandero*'s healing arts come primarily from more recent European and New World sources of the theory and practice of witchcraft, spiritualism, psychic phenomena, and modern medicine, such as the *Grimoire* and the writings of Allen Cardec.

The ideas embodied in medieval and later European witchcraft have contributed heavily to the theoretical base of *curanderismo*. These ideas were constantly reinforced in the popular mind throughout the period of intensive witchhunting that lasted from the early fifteenth century, through its peak around 1600, and into its decline and final disappearance in the early nineteenth century (see Robbins 1959). This coincides with the discovery, conquest, and colonization of the New World, and it can be assumed that these popular concepts accompanied the conquerors. Fortunately, the more ferocious and disgusting practices of the witch burners seem to have been left at home, with the brief exception of the Salem witch trials.

The basic theoretical premise of witchcraft and sorcery is the belief that supernatural forces can be controlled by man himself, rather than their having undisputed control over him. This belief, combined with the teachings of Christianity, creates a dual philosophical system within *curanderismo*. This duality is symbolized by the differences between a religious orientation and a magical orientation. That duality is aptly described by E. A. Hoebel:

> That which distinguishes religion from magic is neither the goodness of one nor the evil of the other, but the state of mind of the believer and his consequent modes of behavior. . . . In the religious state of mind, man acknowledges the superiority of the supernatural powers upon whose action his wellbeing depends. His attitudes are preponderantly those of submission and reverence. . . . The magician, on the other hand, believes that he *controls* supernatural power under certain conditions. He feels confirmed in his belief that if he possesses a tested formula and if he executes it perfectly, barring outside interference, he will get the results which that formula is specified to give. The supernatural power has no volition or choice of its own. It must respond. The magician works with a confidence similar to that of a student in the laboratory who knows that if he follows the manual instructions correctly, he will obtain a pre-

dictable result. The religious attitude and behavior are devout; the magician works with a kind of arrogance— or, at least, self-assurance. [Hoebel 1972 : 578–79]

These philosophies are not necessarily mutually exclusive. They can be and have been combined into a single belief system, where that theoretical system has many flexible facets and is not yet totally integrated into a single theoretical framework. This condition exists in modern scientific medicine, with its official acknowledgement of the physical, psychological, and spiritual components of human health and illness, and its unofficial acknowledgement of the "miracle" of faith. And *curanderismo* shares this theoretical flexibility, although the emphasis placed on the importance of each of these components of the system is somewhat different.

Two closely related concepts from European witchcraft continue to influence modern *curanderismo*. The first is a belief in the existence of a source of supernatural power that can be tapped by human beings who possess the correct incantations, prayers, and rituals. The ingredients used in the spells and the words or even the languages used for the spells may have changed somewhat through time, but many of the rituals used by both *curanderos* (to heal) and *brujos* (to harm) follow the structure of formulas from the Middle Ages and later.

The second is a belief in the ability of some *curanderos* to control or influence spirit beings. Control of spirit beings is exercised through the knowledge of various incantations, prayers, and rituals that can bring about direct human control over spirits. The structure of the spirit-controlling rites is similar to the structure of those designed to tap supernatural power.

One final influence on *curanderismo*, traced to medieval European beliefs about witchcraft and sorcery, has resulted in confusion within the Mexican American community over the ultimate source of the healing power demonstrated by folk healers. One group maintains that the power to heal comes from God; the other group, primarily members of fundamentalist religions, insists that the healing *curandero's* performance is inspired through the power of Satan. This is a traditional dichotomy in Western tradition, as is pointed out by Givry:

> We find the theologians in opposition to the demonists. If cures have taken place at Lourdes or any other sanctuary consecrated by the Church, they are the undeniable work of the Deity. But, similar cures have so taken place in circumstances where the disapproval of the Church has been clearly shown; these cures according to the Church, are the work of the Devil. Hence, the Devil holds in his hands curative powers equal to those of God. [Givry 1971 : 327]

The possibility that the *curandero* may be working through the Devil causes some of the confusion over the moral rightness of seeking help from a proven healer in Mexican American communities. Powerful *curanderos* are restrained from practicing sorcery (antisocial magic) only by their own moral conscience. Each *curandero* has the option of working through good or evil sources, and many people fear them even when seeking their help. There is always the possibility that some spiritual harm may come to the patient even while he is being cured of his malady.

The belief that *curanderos* may be the devil's agents on earth is most pronounced among fundamentalist groups and pentecostal churches. These churches are growing rapidly in Mexican American communities, and their members seem to feel that all works of the folk healers are inspired by the Devil (with or without the knowledge of the healer). They quote appropriate passages from the Bible that demonstrate that the Devil is loose in the world and that these works (the healings) are the kind the Devil uses to subvert mankind by performing miracles. This attitude, combined with a fear of the unknown, and perhaps unknowable, source of the *curandero*'s power produces confusion about the morality of using the *curandero*'s services. The more powerful *curanderos* publicly admit that both good and evil sources of power are available to them, a fact that increases their reputations but does nothing to allay doubts about the morality of their calling.

Some of the most recent influences on *curanderismo* arise from the writings of the eighteenth-, nineteenth-, and twentieth-century European spiritualists and psychic researchers. The growing importance of the scientific method during the last few centuries, and the end of persecution for witchcraft, touched off intensive and wide-ranging investigations of the validity of ghosts, spirits, mediums, fortune tellers, telekinesis, and a hundred other psychic phenomena. Most of this research was anecdotal, with occasional exceptions such as the work done at the Rhine Institute at Duke University. Most researchers have been content to pile one report, one case, one anecdote on top of another in the hope that others will be convinced of the validity of psychic phenomena. Other writers have ignored the necessity for proof altogether by assuming these phenomena exist and have devoted their energies to sharing their knowledge with the other adepts through the reporting of ancient sources of knowledge or through writing of their own experiences and knowledge gained from direct experimentation (see Huson 1970). The publication of such works has created an enormous volume of information, misinformation, and speculation that is currently available to the general public and to believers. One result has been the spread of both spiritualist and psychic healers from Europe to the United States and Mexico.

The most influential spiritualist writer is Allen Kardec, who is directly responsible for the recent rapid growth of "spiritual temples" in Mexican American communities. Kardec has produced a series of works that explain the structure, maintenance, and function of spiritual healing centers and provide careful descriptions of the rituals, prayers, and incantations necessary to the temple ceremonies (see Kardec 1970).

Another important spiritualist movement is based on the life, teachings, and spirit of a famous young folk healer (now dead) from northern Mexico, el Niño Fidencio. The *Fidencistas* have built large temples in several Mexican cities, with smaller ones scattered around Mexico and the United States (including Chicago). These *centros* are staffed by trance mediums who, often in flower-decked rooms, don purple robes, go into trance, and (in their words) let the spirit of el Niño descend on them, their bodies forming a link between the material and spiritual realms of existence. Through this linkage, the immortal spirit of el Niño performs cures, does consultations, even predicts the outcome of future events for the members of his cult.

Spiritualist healing is now taught in *centros espiritistas* in Mexico and by traveling adepts from these *centros*, as well as by local adepts. Many professional *curanderos* state that today many imporant parts of their healing knowledge come through spiritual training (*desarrollo*) and subsequent contact with the spiritual realm. They claim some of their cures are done through the use of spiritual knowledge that simply comes into their minds or comes from spiritual voices (*las voces*), while other cures are carried out directly through the agency of spirits themselves. These spirits are those who have agreed to aid the *curandero* in his or her work.

The phenomenon of psychic healing is also becoming more common among *curanderos*. It is said to be performed by the *curandero* directing psychic energies (*corrientes mentales*) directly at the afflicted organ—a form of mind over matter. The importance of psychic healing to the theories held by *curanderos* is rapidly growing, especially in urban areas.

The effects of the medical knowledge, beliefs, and practices of American Indian groups on *curanderismo* have varied significantly from area to area. The most important influence in all areas was the impact that the incredibly rich and extensive knowledge of medicinal herbs existing in Native American groups has had on European pharmacology. One of the first tasks undertaken by individuals in expeditions to the New World was to discover and classify new plants and animals, making careful note of their medicinal properties (see Foster 1953:203). The lack of sufficient doctors and medical facilities in the New World caused books about these newly discovered medicinal herbs, along with their Old World counterparts, to be disseminated throughout Mexico, especially in the frontier regions. The direct descendants of these books are still widely used by both Mexican and Mexican American housewives (see Arias n.d., Capo n.d., and Wagner n.d.).

The most important of the early botanical books and medical compendiums, according to anthropologist Margaritta Kay (1974a, 1974b), was the *Florilegio Medicinal*, a three-volume set encompassing medicine, surgery, and pharmacology. Written by a Jesuit lay brother, Juan de Esteyneffer (Esteyneffer 1711), this work had a lasting effect on the practices of folk medicine along the northern frontier areas of New Spain.

The work of the 16th century natural historians of Mexico had already been incorporated into the knowledge of the European apothecary. These included Hernandez (via Ximinez 1615) who had been sent by Philip II of Spain to report on the *materia medica* available in New Spain, and Nicolas Monardes, the Spanish physician, who wrote knowledgeably about these herbs without ever leaving Spain. Sahagun's data were not available until

1829, but his influence was felt through Martin de la Cruz and Juan Badianus, who produced the beautiful Badianus manuscript of 1595 in which indigenous herbs are given humoral classification (see Guerra n.d. and 1961). For Esteyneffer, the most important writer of this kind was Farfan (see Comas 1954). [Kay 1974a: 10]

Farfan, mentioned in the above quote, had written a book in 1592, *Tractado Breve de Medicina* (Farfan 1944) to aid the poor and people in rural areas by providing them with remedies and cures from both New and Old World medicinal herbs (Kay 1974a: 11). This book may have inspired Esteyneffer to produce his own larger treatise on the same subject.

The *Florilegio Medicinal*, through Esteyneffer's teaching efforts among the Jesuits in the missions of northwestern Mexico, is at least partly responsible for the blending of Old and New World cures for many of the folk diseases and other illnesses recognized by Mexican Americans throughout the southwestern United States. It is also responsible for similar beliefs and practices among such different American Indian groups as the Papago, Pima, Yaqui, PaiPai, Tarahumara, and Tepehuan, among whom the Jesuits also had missions (Kay 1974b).

Nentuig (unknown 1951: 43) spoke of the "old Spanish women who have either set themselves up or have become in the natural course of the events the College of Physicians of Sonora." I think they used the *Florilegio Medicinal*, which compiled the herbal lore of various Indians of the Southwest, combined it with the *materia medica* of Europe, attached them to disease conditions that were scientifically recognized in the eighteenth century and diffused this knowledge throughout the Northwest of Mexico and the Southwest United States. For *pasmo, alferecia, empacho, mollera caida, tirisia*

1 *pujos*, which have first been explained by Es-
ᴄᴄyneffer and are still diagnosed today, are cured by the
same herbs. [Kay 1974b:8]

Other bits of information were added to the immense
herbal knowledge of *curanderismo* through direct contact
with various American Indian groups, and through individual experimentation on the part of the Spanish settlers in
the northern frontier areas. The fact that access to modern
medical services is still limited by poverty, isolation, and
discrimination in south Texas has encouraged the use of
this herbal knowledge up to the present.

The other influences that Native American folk medicine
has had on *curanderismo* are more difficult to isolate. In
many of the border areas, such as the Lower Rio Grande Valley of Texas, the environment supported only scattered
groups of hunters and gatherers before the influx of the
Spanish. Thus, the amount of contact between settlers and
Indian groups was far less than between the conquerors and
the larger agriculturally based Indian populations in Mexico
and parts of South America. In the Southwestern Pueblo Indian complex, where greater contact might have been possible, these exchanges were limited by suppression of Native
American beliefs and activities and secrecy on the part of
the Indians. Further Native American influences may be revealed to be a part of *curanderismo* as more research is done
in this area, but as of now Mexican American folk medicine
seems to have primarily a European historical and theoretical base.

Until the development of extensive irrigation works in
the early 1900s, most of the southwestern United States was
best suited for ranching and very small scale farming. People
lived on scattered homesteads, isolated from the medical resources of the cities. Very few health-care professionals
were attracted to the area because of the lack of facilities,
small population, and the immense distances. Herbs, pray-

ers, and faith in the *curandero*'s healing ability were often the only medical resources these people had to combat either illness or accident.

Urban centers grew as irrigation works were developed. These towns and cities were progressively linked by roads, telegraph, railroads, and other communication systems tying the Southwest more directly into the political and economic centers of the United States. Previously the region had been isolated or had been more directly linked to northern Mexican towns than to centers in the United States. New concentrations of people in the Southwest, and the wealth associated with the agricultural and mineral industries being developed, have attracted growing numbers of doctors, nurses, and medical services to the area. Thus modern medical practices began to influence the practice of *curanderos* in areas like the Lower Rio Grande Valley. Yet even after modern medicine became established in the area, poverty, discrimination, prejudice, and cultural barriers to communication and understanding combined to deny many Mexican Americans access to the new medical system. For these excluded people the *curanderos* continued to provide the best available care.

Today *curanderos* in urbanized areas like south Texas recognize and accept the diagnosis of many, if not most, diseases defined by Western medicine. Some even use modern drugs, anatomical charts, and clinical facilities that closely resemble a doctor's office (Alger 1974: 283–84) in their own practices. More commonly they simply recognize conventional categories of disease and refer patients to doctors for those diseases which modern medicine has proven highly successful in healing. In addition, they recognize certain diseases that mimic, for instance, tuberculosis, asthma, and cancer, but are thought to be caused by magical works placed on the patient by *brujos*.

Since the return of World War II veterans, more and more Mexican Americans have gained entrance into the mainstream of American society, including its medical system. However, too many people are still very poor, even though there is a growing middle and upper class made up mainly of businessmen and professionals. The result of this change is that some Mexican American patients now make use of both *curanderismo* and modern medicine. We shall now consider why people prefer one system to the other or, more commonly, use both simultaneously.

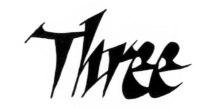

THE CULTURAL
CONTEXT
OF ILLNESS

A MAN IN SOUTH TEXAS and a man in Saudi Arabia will both
have the same general biological needs when they contract
tuberculosis. But their physical needs must be met in ways
that take into account the existing differences in their social systems (differences in customs, beliefs, family structure, religion, and economic class) and their expectations of
health care and health personnel. The best way practitioners
can successfully treat the whole person is to understand the
social framework that surrounds his biological illness.

Differences in the social framework of illness come about
through the ways different cultural groups are taught to label reality, mark time, and use space. Labels break down reality into manageable categories. Objects, ideas, emotions,
and relationships are grouped together or separated from one
another for special emphasis in each culture. The world
view, the communication, and perception of reality in any
two cultures is different since no two languages categorize
reality in exactly the same way. Perception is further inten-
sified or directed by differences in the use of time and space
in different cultural systems.

The interpretation of disease and illness, which includes
both health-belief systems and rehabilitation procedures, is
bound to culture. Culture teaches the individual to interpret

pain in terms that are meaningful to him as an individual and as a member of a group. A member of one culture may believe his stomach is upset because he ate too fast, so he takes an Alka-Seltzer, while someone in another culture may believe his stomach is hot, so he takes a refreshing herb. In one culture being ill may mean dispensation from responsibility, while in another culture it may be an open admission of weakness.

The Mexican American cultural framework acknowledges the existence of two sources of illness, one natural and one supernatural. The natural source is recognized and treated by modern medicine and *curanderos;* the supernatural source is recognized and treated by *curanderos* alone. Given this double perspective, any particular illness can come from either source. The sick person may have identical symptoms regardless of which source instigated the disease. Natural diseases are cured by herbs, drugs, surgery, or other scientific medical techniques. The failure of these techniques is one indication that the illness is caused by a *trabajo* (spell) and requires treatment by a *curandero* to remove the causal agent of the disease. Successful treatment of the illness by the *curandero* is taken as further proof that supernatural causation of illness actually exists and promotes the persistence of this dual framework. *Curanderos,* however, do not use magic alone. They also treat physical illnesses by the use of herbs, poultices, massages, and other traditional procedures.

The family, as the main socialization unit for many health beliefs, teaches its members how to tell whether an illness exists. It is through the family that a child learns to interpret his reality. Part of this reality is learning certain health habits and health practices (for example, brushing teeth, keeping the body clean, eating proper foods, playing in safe areas, and learning how to cross the street). One child may learn that it is important to clean and nurse a cut, while another may learn that it is shameful to cry when he is hurt.

Different cultures encourage different responses to illness. This socialization process remains as a permanent part of a person's knowledge and will ultimately guide his health behavior.

Mexican American families are not unlike other families in socializing children in health concepts and health practices. They encourage concepts and beliefs held by the community. An informant tells how she learned about *curanderos* as a child:

> When I was a child I used to hear my family talking. Someone placed something on my father and he got very ill. He almost died. Other things happened to other members of our family, but they died because they did not get cured. They were given something to eat and their bellies got big and hard. The rest of their bodies sort of withered down.

Another informant who is very knowledgeable in the use of herbs tells how she acquired her skill:

> Well, it is that one learns these things because of grandparents, aunts, and from experience. . . . Both my grandmothers healed with herbs. Since I was small, I was very interested in knowing this. I paid much attention. My father likes to have many herbs at home, to cure. He also told me many things.

The family usually decides whether an illness is likely to become critical, and the family ordinarily begins the treatment. In purely practical terms, any serious illness will upset most families. However, it is the cultural interpretation of the illness which will define what health resources are needed and what health practitioner will be consulted. Ease of access frequently determines whether or how often a patient seeks medical help, and what sort of help he seeks.

The first problem of access to medical care for Mexican Americans is economic. The family's access to modern medical services depends largely on its income. Other forms of health-care delivery—county hospitals, public health clinics, migrant clinics—involve a series of complicated bureaucratic procedures which discourage people from these services or, through their regulations, leave some people without access. This bureaucratic entanglement is unfortunate, since these mostly federal programs have been devised to try and overcome the economic barrier to providing health care, and have succeeded for some groups within the community. However, the piecemeal development and application of these programs, combined with an overall lack of coordination, has led to continued fragmentation of medical systems for the poor in the Lower Rio Grande Valley. The impersonality and insensitivity of bureaucracies is a problem for all people, but it may be especially trying for Mexican Americans, who place high values on personal relationships and a personal approach to life. Inconveniences (like filling out forms, waiting, and going to different doctors for different illnesses and to different clinics on different days for different members of the family) can be and sometimes are avoided by calling on the services of the *curandero* instead.

Historically, traditional folk medicine, rather than modern medicine, has been the main resource for Mexican American families. Agricultural isolation, poverty, discrimination, respect for age and for experience, and strong traditions made people rely mainly on themselves and their own resources to maintain their health and take care of their sick. As Mexican Americans became more urban, they came into closer contact with modern medicine. They learned to rely on modern medicine without giving up their own traditional medicine, which has no bureaucracy and is closer personally and culturally. Thus Mexican Americans in south Texas have what might be considered a dual orientation toward health care.

A growing number of studies on popular medical beliefs,

folk medicine, and non-Western medicine has demonstrated that the scientific medical framework is often very different from other existing frameworks of health and health care (see Fabrega 1970). The germ theory of disease is important within scientific medical theories, while social and moral conditions are not frequently seen as direct causal agents of illness. The reverse is true for many other cultural perceptions of illness. In other cultures, including a number of Western religious groups, moral lapses or social wrongdoing is thought to bring about illness, and sickness is seen as a punishment from God.

Curanderismo, as an alternative system of health care, places a strong emphasis on the social, psychological, and spiritual factors contributing to illness and poor health. In the first place, the work of a *curandero* is sanctioned by the community where he practices. Second, most healing procedures involve an evaluation of a patient's family and support system (for example, co-workers, friends, and schoolmates). Third, there is always the ritual petition to God or other spiritual beings to help with the healing process. The spiritual factors involved in *curanderismo* are beyond the normal limits of social science. However, we cannot deny that the violation of certain moral codes and the development of guilt complexes do constitute threats to good health. In the same vein, once a person becomes ill, faith can become an important factor in his recovery. That social and moral disruptions can produce physical problems is illustrated by this report from one of our informants:

When my twins were born fifteen years ago, this lady who rented one of my houses was very close to me. She would come over for coffee and we would talk. I used to help her with food and clothing. She had a very large family. Then suddenly one day she left. The house was empty. She owed me for the rent and other things. Shortly after that I began to feel sick. I felt like rubber, as

if my whole body were a sponge. My mother-in-law consulted with this lady in McAllen. She said that this
neighbor had harmed me. We searched in the empty
house and we found the harm [*el dano*]. It was a crucifix.
They had taken off the Christ and tied it with red ribbons, wire, and herbs.

According to this informant the *curandero* attending the
case was able to perform a ritual that destroyed the harm (*el
dano*), restored harmony to her social environment by pun-
ishing her former neighbor, and restored our informant to
health.

Frameworks for beliefs about illness are so diverse that serious problems can result when a person believing in one
framework is being treated by a person who believes in another framework. For Mexican Americans, this conflict has
occasionally led to the incorrect diagnosis of serious psychological disturbance. Karno (1965:2) describes a case where
obviously the patient's symptoms had one meaning within
her own cultural framework but were evaluated differently
by a health care professional from another culture:

When Josephine Martinez was 31 and had been married
for 10 years, she visited a psychiatric clinic. She com-
plained of feeling increasingly depressed, nervous,
introverted and shy. During her marriage she had become
plagued by fears and extreme irritability. Mrs. Martinez'
parents were born in Mexico and until beginning a Los
Angeles public school, she had spoken only Spanish. Her
earliest feelings and beliefs were steeped in the rural
Mexican folk culture of her parents. In the psychiatric
clinic a skilled clinical psychologist made the following
remark concerning Mrs. Martinez' psychological test results: "Her thought processes are somewhat confused
and illogical to the point of bizarreness at times. She said
'true' to an MMPI item about being possessed by evil
spirits. . . ." Based on this and other information, the

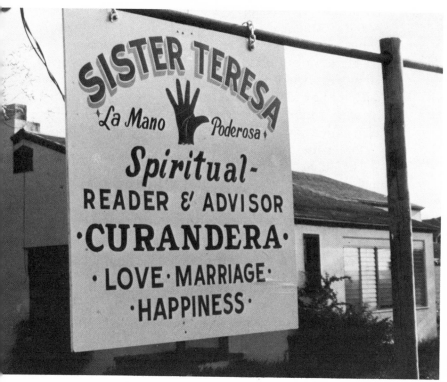

Sign outside a *curandera*'s house

psychologist made the diagnosis of "early schizophrenic reaction." Clinical interviews in the course of treatment revealed a moderately depressed woman with strong motivation for help, but no signs of the psychosis "elicited" by psychological testing.

In traditional Mexican American culture, feelings of depression are often interpreted as spiritual weakness. Spiritual weakness often leads to temptation and harassment by other spirits which may want to harm a person. This view is not unlike fundamental Catholic beliefs. Moreover, the idea that spirits are close at hand and can directly influence the health and well-being of a person is not bizarre to some Mexican Americans. Therefore, the indigenous disease categories of a society and the attitudes and expectations of its people toward healing and healers must be recognized as factors that promote communication or misunderstanding between provider and patient. The ability to identify disease categories from the patient's perspective can allow health-care professionals to make culturally appropriate responses to local patterns.

The differences in world view between the professional and the patient are vividly illustrated by the differences in their theories about illness. The modern medical framework recognizes two broad categories of diseases: those which are primarily physiological and those which are primarily social-psychological in origin. The medical system directs most of its effort and emphasis toward the physiological. "To the scientifically trained physician . . . an illness usually implies a set of molecular, biochemical, and physiological processes or events. Illnesses are grouped by him in terms of cause, organ system affected and/or pathological processes" (Fabrega 1971:25).

This emphasis on the biological aspects of illness has numerous effects on its treatment. Whenever a sick person comes into the modern health-care system, he is normally given a series of tests that are designed to determine which physiological disorder is causing the symptoms. With the exception of obvious mental disturbances, only after the possibility of physical causation has been ruled out is any serious attention paid to the psychological status of the patient. Social factors as causes of ill health are virtually ignored.

More recently, another problem has been added to the physiological orientation of modern medicine. In order to cope with vast amounts of new knowledge and increasingly complicated technical skills, the modern medical system has developed more and more specializations. In many cases this approach to medicine has changed the "isolated individual" to the "fragmented individual." The occasional patient who confronts the medical system with two or more diseases, especially if they affect different organ systems, may have two or more specialists treating him at the same time. The efficiency of the hospital is also increased by grouping patients with common needs, so this patient's separate treatments may be conducted in altogether different facilities. This type of treatment, through its emphasis on the particular problem of a diseased organism, tends to fragment the health professional's perception of the patient as a whole. Fragmentation increases problems in communication and understanding among the specialists themselves, who may out of necessity be giving the patient conflicting advice. Specialization undoubtedly produces the most efficient treatment of specific diseases but makes it very difficult to treat the whole patient.

Friedson (1970:59), among others, sees this specialized approach to illness as an extension of the "common-sense individualism" of Western society. The patient's social framework—his family ties, friends, work, religion, and community, plus the cultural definitions of illness he learned at home—makes it impossible for him to think of himself as an isolated or fragmented individual. The practitioner's framework makes it nearly impossible to think of the patient as anything else. Neither of these frameworks can be considered completely wrong or completely right in any ultimate sense. They are different perceptions of the same basic reality of illness, which can cause problems in curing that illness.

Mexican Americans share the larger society's perspective of health and illness. In addition, for many Mexican Americans *curanderismo* forms part of an ever-present pattern of cultural choices. Health-care professionals (especially some monolingual, monocultural Anglos) are often unaware or insensitive to a Mexican American's ability to move comfortably in two cultures. Mexican Americans have a choice of two languages, two types of food, two lifestyles, and two health-care systems. This cultural switching is so natural that it disrupts neither thought nor social processes.

Most people choose their system of health care on the basis of comfort, economics, and accessibility. Some Mexican Americans would never go to a *curandero*, and others completely reject the modern health-care system. However, since both systems offer something to individual and family needs, for many Mexican Americans the choice between *curanderismo* and modern medicine is not an either/or proposition. Some persons use both systems, taking advantage of the benefits of each. For example, a mother of seven small children explains why she uses both the *curandero* and the physician:

> We are very peculiar (*curiosos*). If I know that I am sick, if I have a heart problem or high blood pressure, I'll go see the doctor. I also take my children . . . vaccinations, throat infections, or whatever. Sometimes you go, and the doctor gives you a shot, and you still don't get well. When the doctor can't help me then I go see [a healer]. Sometimes I go to him first. He gives good treatments. I am able to save the doctor's fee. We sort of make ourselves fit wherever we can (*donde quiera nos acomodamos*).

A woman in her late thirties who suffers from rheumatism gives the following account:

> I went to the doctor. He made me get undressed and put on a little robe. He examined my hands and my knees. Then he told me I had rheumatism. I already knew that! He said he couldn't do anything for me, just give me a shot. He charged me fifteen dollars; now I go to him only when I feel real sick and need the drugs. Otherwise I go see [a healer]. I don't know why but I have more confidence and faith in him. He gives me herbs, and I feel

fine. However, when I feel fine for a long time, I stop taking the herbs. Then I get sick all over again.

Mexican Americans have been expected to move away from traditional medicine as they become more urban and more educated. Their socialization process, however, instills certain beliefs about health and health care and certain values regarding the behavior of individuals. The Mexican American socialization process calls for warm interpersonal relationships, especially in times of stress and crisis, when the primary group (family and its support system) must come together to solve or at least ameliorate the problem. This person-centered aspect and emphasis places more importance on personality and quality of interaction than on the diplomas and fancy equipment displayed in an office. At least in the Lower Rio Grande Valley, *curanderismo* has an obvious advantage over modern medicine in interpersonal relationships, and *curanderos* continue to draw large numbers of people.

Based on their own subjective criteria of what is considered to be the best or the most convenient, Mexican American families often make use of both traditional and modern medicine. The *curandero* and the physician are often colleagues, unknown to each other and working at different levels. The physician works to rehabilitate the patient's body, and the *curandero* works to reintegrate him with his family and his community. Alternate health resources make up the health-care environment of south Texas and provide the Mexican American community with a variety of services.

Most Mexican American housewives in the Lower Rio Grande Valley are familiar with a number of *remedios caseros* (home remedies) as well as useful patent medicines (such as aspirin, epsom salts, and baby powder) and first-aid techniques. All of these are used as a first line of defense against common health problems encountered in every home. This type of healing is probably the most common form in all cultures, and, as with other kinds of healing systems, some people show a special aptitude for it. They gain enough knowledge of the subject to be considered especially good at healing, perhaps even experts, by their circle of acquaintances. Some individuals even go beyond a general knowledge of healing to actual specializations.

A whole set of specializations exists within *curanderismo* in south Texas. These practices offer Mexican Americans a wide variety of services, some perhaps unique to the border area and others probably found in most Mexican American *barrios*. The specializations described below are a convenient catalog of the types of healing that go on in the *barrios*, from the point of view of the social scientist and of many members of the community. However, they should not be taken as necessarily reflecting the healers' own perspectives on healing. The knowledge of many of the *curanderos* in the Lower Rio Grande Valley encompasses two or more of these specializations. Finally, the descriptions are meant more as an indication of the breadth of the communities' self-help resources than an exhaustive catalog of all the practices within *curanderismo*.

Most visible and most widely used are the *parteras* (midwives), *sobadores* (who treat muscle sprains), *yerberos* (herbalists), the *señoras* who read cards, and the individuals whom we are calling *curanderos*, professional healers who know and use the theoretical system presented in this study and who heal full time, seeing from five to sixty patients a day.

The idea of specializations is somewhat misleading, even though it provides a useful approach to describing the practices within the folk-healing system. One problem is that many of the healers in south Texas practice or have knowledge of more than one of these special areas. Another is that these specializations do not correspond directly to the theoretical structure of *curanderismo*, as would more nearly be the case for modern medicine. Nevertheless, these specializations are common enough to necessitate their description as a part of the total folk-healing environment.

One of the most visible specializations of folk medicine in the Lower Rio Grande Valley is *parteras* (midwives). In Texas, "assisting in the delivery of a child" has been deliberately excluded from the Medical Practices Act. Although legislation is frequently proposed to regulate midwifery, so far the only legal requirements are that each birth be recorded at the county courthouse and that silver nitrate drops be placed in the newborn's eyes. Literally anyone can be a midwife in Texas, and the border areas of south Texas abound in midwives. More than thirty were contacted in the course of our research over the past four years. *Parteras* delivered approximately one out of every five babies in the valley (2,419 live births out of 11,828) in 1978. The highest percentage of these births occurred in Brownsville, but no fewer than 10 percent were recorded in Hidalgo County.

Several factors contribute to the demand for *parteras'* services. Poverty-level incomes cause many women to make use of *parteras* rather than medical doctors or registered nurse-midwives. Some local doctors have made an effort to provide free services for these women, but the large number of families with poverty-level incomes, the frequency of births in these families, and the recognized scarcity of doctors in the area, make this admirable effort an impossible task. The patient's choice, then, is normally between a combined doctor and hospital fee of $700 or more, and a $200 fee for *partera* services on the United States side of the border or an $80 fee on the Mexican side for those close enough to utilize this service. The doctor's and hospital's fees normally represent an impossibly large proportion of the family income, especially when tied into the necessity of putting up a deposit of $250 or more before entry into the hospital system. Since over 50 percent of the families in the valley fall below federal poverty levels, the *parteras* often become the only viable choice for the delivery of a baby.

Mexican Americans are not the only users of the *parteras'* services. Many people from low-income families in Mexico view entry into the United States as a possible escape from their poverty. Therefore, many of the infants delivered by *parteras* in the border areas are the children of Mexican nationals, who see the child's automatic citizenship as a legal bridge into the U.S. The hospitals in the valley strongly discourage those who cannot meet their entrance requirements (for instance, their required deposit) from using their services, including the emergency room. The patient's recourse is to local *parteras* or to waiting outside the hospital until the baby is crowning, at which point the hospital cannot send them back across the border. Most women choose *parteras*.

Some women seek the services of *parteras* by simple cultural preference. The *partera* is female, thereby protecting traditional ideas of modesty that are sometimes strained by the presence of a male doctor. The *partera* is usually a relative or friend; it is highly unlikely that the *partera* and patient are completely unknown to one another. This produces trust between them and often improves the patient's state of mind during the delivery. Finally, no barriers exist to communication between patient and practitioner. They not only share the same language, they share the same vocabulary, values, and sociocultural background. Thus, for some families the *partera* becomes a part of family tradition and is seen as a culturally appropriate alternative to delivering in the hospital.

Of the three factors, the first two are currently the strongest contributors to the persistence of *parteras* in south Texas, although the third could become increasingly important if the valley follows the national trend toward home delivery.

One indication of the availability of *parteras* in the valley is that many of them advertise in the Yellow Pages. Some have gotten together to set up group practices that allow them a regular night off. Some give prenatal care and postnatal checkups and advice. Many are affiliated with physicians and refer difficult cases to them. Some of these women also act as *curanderas*, but this seems somewhat rare. In fact, the *parteras* appeared to us to be the least concerned with magic and sorcery of all of the folk healers. Some used herbal teas to speed contractions or ease pain, but very few invoked any supernatural assistance.

Earlier researchers in the valley (for example, Madsen 1964) identified a group of healers called *hueseros* (bone setters). They were responsible for setting bones and dealing with sprains and muscle pulls. They no longer exist as a group, their function having been taken over by modern medical facilities and osteological specialists. However, since chiropractors are relatively rare in the valley, part of the *hueseros'* functions have been taken over by a group called *sobadores*.

Sobadores are individuals who have a *don* for treating sore muscles, sprains, tenseness, and so on. They treat by massaging, rubbing, or kneading the affected part of the body. Our informants indicated that they distinguish two different types of treatment, the *mesaje* and the *sobadita*. A *mesaje* is a general massage that is performed for a person who is suffering pain or headaches due to nervous tension. It is aimed at relaxing the patient and removing the tenseness. The *sobadita* is a treatment for a specific muscle problem like sprained ankle or a cramp.

The *sobadores* do not have formal training, but they often follow a set procedure in the treatment. The *mesajes* are normally straightforward. The patients come to the *sobadores* and request treatment, which is given. The *sobaditas* require more elaborate knowledge and precautions. One informant stated that she examines the injured area and if there is an indication of a broken bone, she sends the client to the hospital. She also never massages an area that is badly swollen. Instead she treats it with a warm epsom-salt soak to reduce the swelling and afterwards manipulates the damaged area to help it heal. She often uses olive oil when she is giving a massage.

During the fall, many of the *sobadores'* patients are young high-school students with football injuries. At other times the clientele ranges from young children to old people seeking relief from arthritis. At the time of the research, the *sobadores* were charging about three dollars for their treatments, much less than either chiropractors or physicians.

Nearly every town in south Texas, regardless of its size, has a store called a *yerberia* or a *botica*. This shop stocks herbs, perfumes, oils, candles, and much of the other paraphernalia used both by housewives and by folk healers. Many of the housewives in south Texas grow common herbs in their yards to treat childhood and common adult ailments. In addition, there are a few individuals with a special talent for working with herbal remedies. These people know literally hundreds of herbal treatments. They grow some of the herbs, such as *manzanilla* (camomile) for colic or *yerba buena* (mint) for stomachaches. Other herbs they purchase from the *boticas* and *yerberias*. One such herb is *habas de San Ignacio* (the seed of the monkey dinner bell tree) that is used to stop excessive drinking (see Trotter and Chavira 1978). Some of them use the books published in Mexico (for example, Wagner n.d. or Capo n.d.) on herbs. Since the use of herbs is an important part of *curanderismo*, more extensive information on the use of herbal remedies is provided in chapter 5.

One group of specialists in the valley is the women who use cards to console clients, predict the future, and explain past occurrences. Nearly every *curandero* contacted had some knowledge of the use of cards to diagnose particular problems; however, the card-reading specialists make such practices their entire avocation. One informant had a clientele of approximately fifty women students from Pan American University. She specialized in helping women of that particular age. Other readers had much more mixed client populations. Unlike the stereotyped gypsy fortuneteller, these *señoras* make specific predictions, normally in three areas: health, home life, and social condition (including legal and business matters).

The patient-reader encounter is similar to most such interactions. The client approaches the reader, often being brought by another client. They chat socially for a while and then the reading begins. Three different decks of cards are used by the *señoras*. Most use the forty-card Mexican deck with figures of gold coins, clubs, swords, and cups on them. A few use the fifty-two-card deck that is popular in the United States, with its stylized hearts, diamonds, spades, and coverleaf-shaped club pattern. And a very few use the tarot deck. The three decks are thought to have increasingly detailed predictive and diagnostic capabilities, starting with the Mexican deck and working up to the tarot deck.

Sometimes the client is asked to shuffle the cards while thinking of a specific question that is to be answered. At other times the reader shuffles the cards. The cards are shuffled a specific (magical) number of times, such as three, seven, or eleven. They are then cut, normally into three piles, by the client. The three cards exposed by the cuts are read to set the general orientation of the card reading. Then the reader begins arranging all of the cards into sets. Each set is a particular shape, such as a square, a cross, a triangle, a rectangle, a pyramid, or a shape like a pitchfork, called the Devil's trident. The reading is given in stages, called *tendidas* by one informant. Each *tendida* provides information about home, health, and social conditions. If a reading consists of more than one *tendida*, the later stages are used to confirm the information of the earlier *tendidas*, and to provide additional details about them. Each card has a particular meaning, but those meanings are expanded upon, modified, or strengthened by the surrounding cards or by particular combinations of cards.

During the normal reading, the reader both gives and gets information. Much of the reading consists of the reader's telling· the client what has happened and what is going to happen to him. This information is given in a very authoritative manner. When one client told a reader that something the señora had detailed as having happened had not in fact occurred, the *curandera* replied that it had happened, and the client just had not noticed. Specific details, such as dates, places, names, and detailed descriptions of individuals are not uncommon in readings. Clients are often asked for confirmation of these details, and when it is given the reader appears to gain confidence and the client's satisfaction with the reading and rapport with the reader increases in direct proportion. It was not uncommon for informants to tell the authors that the reader had provided them with intimate details about their past lives to which he or she had no known access. Other informants told of going to two or more readers and receiving identical predictions, which had subsequently come true. The continuing occurrence of these events, regardless of how they are produced by the readers, guarantees a clientele for them into the forseeable future.

The term *curandero* literally means "healer," from the Spanish verb *curar* ("to heal"). Therefore, anyone who performs any type of healing, from brain surgery to psychic surgery, could theoretically be called a *curandero*. However, the term is normally used in the literature to denote a folk healer as opposed to a member of the modern medical system. Even this restriction, however, leaves far too many areas of confusion, because of the numerous services Mexican American folk healers perform and because of the looseness with which the term has been used in describing various types of folk healers in the social-science literature.

There are distinct differences in the practice of *curanderismo* in various geographical areas of the United States, and some confusion in interpreting *curanderismo* has been

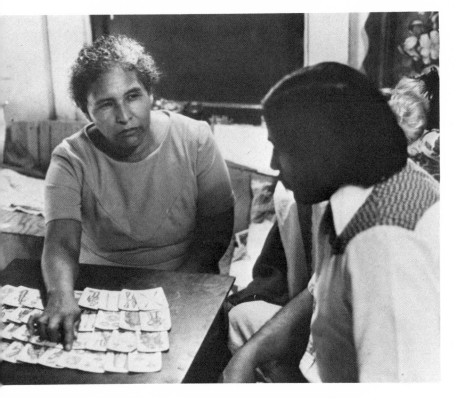

Curandera instructing an apprentice in the reading of cards

produced by these differences. In part, this is due to geographical and historical differences between Hispanic communities in the United States. *Curanderos* have had to modify their beliefs and practices to fit existing environmental and social conditions within their communities, just as medical scientists in other areas of the world have had to do. One cannot expect that the health conditions of a population would be exactly the same in a desert, in a jungle, or on a high mountain plateau. As people settled different ecological zones, they accumulated medical practices that were necessary to the special character of the environment and discarded some that were no longer useful. They also maintained many practices that were important and persistent parts of their cultural system, practices that maintained their significance in all environments because of their linkage to the community's overall needs or to central cultural themes.

While many of these specialists are called *curanderos* by the public, we have decided to use the term somewhat more specifically. When used as a *generic* term in the rest of this work, the term will refer to an individual with particular characteristics. They are recognized by themselves and by their community as having a special ability to heal. The *don* is the basic difference between the healer and the nonhealer, especially with regard to the practice of the supernatural aspects of *curanderismo*. In addition, the term *curandero* applies to individuals who are aware of and make use of the theoretical knowledge of *curanderismo*. Finally, *curanderos* are individuals who heal on a regular, often fulltime basis and who see an average of five or more patients a day. These three criteria are used to distinguish between professional healers and laymen who use some part of the available knowledge in folk medicine. We shall describe the theoretical system used by the professionals.

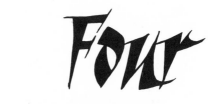

CURANDEROS'
THEORIES
OF HEALING

CURANDEROS IN SOUTH TEXAS explain their abilities to heal and describe their healing techniques by referring to three levels of treatment. The levels are the material (*nivel material*), the spiritual (*nivel espiritual*) and the mental (*nivel mental*). They are not mutually exclusive, in that a *curandero* can have the gift (*don*) for working on one, two, or all three levels. The levels are also similar in treating problems of a physical nature and of social and psychological disorders. However, each level necessitates a different gift (*don*), the training techniques are somewhat different, and each level is thought to tap a different aspect of supernatural power. The *curanderos* recognize two types of illnesses, the natural (primarily physical but also psychosocial) and the supernatural, and they claim to have the resources necessary to treat both.

Natural illnesses are described by the *curanderos* as illnesses caused by natural agents rather than supernatural agents. Many *curanderos* recognize a variety of illnesses that are identical to those categories of illness recognized by physicians. Examples of these are hypertension, diabetes, tuberculosis, senile psychosis, and mental retardation. When faced by natural illnesses, *curanderos* often recommend the services of physicians to their patients, and they seek the physician's services for themselves. Other natural illnesses recognized by *curanderos* are those which have a humoral etiology. One such illness is *bilis*, a folk illness brought about by excessive and prolonged anger and fear. When someone is in this condition, the *curanderos* say that excessive bitter bile flows into the person's system, causing him to become tense and irritable, to lose his appetite, and in some cases to suffer migraine headaches. Another example of a humoral illness is colic, which is sometimes believed to be caused by an excessive coldness in the victim's stomach. In this case a warm herb ("warm" in the humoral classification) such as *manzanilla* is given to restore the natural balance of the humors in the patient's body, thereby bringing relief.

Other illnesses which *curanderos* recognize and treat are those which have been brought about by supernatural means—by sorcerers or malevolent spirits, for example. The existence of these supernatural forces is explained by the *curanderos* in various ways. Some *curanderos* believe in the existence of two universal "minds" or "powers" or even supernatural beings, such as God and the Devil—one positive and good, one negative and evil—which are capable of influencing the destiny of human beings. These *curanderos* see themselves as being able to tap the power of both of these universal forces to harm or heal another individual. This they do through the manipulation of the knowledge they have of the material, spiritual, or psychic levels of healing.

The simplest and most common gift of healing among *curanderos* is the ability to work on the material level. An individual working on the material level (*trabajando en lo material*) is said to be working while awake as opposed to being in trance. Healers working on this level use numerous objects and rituals to effect cures. The objects include herbs, patent medicines, common household items (eggs, lemons, garlic, and ribbon, for example), and religious or mystical symbols (water, oils, incense, perfumes, and so forth). The ceremonies include prayers, ritual sweepings or cleansings (*barridas* or *limpias*), and other complex rituals using all or some of the special objects. For physical ailments the herbs alone are often considered sufficient to bring about a cure. For psychological, spiritual, or magical problems, the *curanderos* frequently combine the herbs, objects, and rituals into a special cure (*curación*) designed to eliminate a specific problem.

On the material level, the objects (tools) and rituals are used in prescribed, preset formulas designed to bring about the desired results. This is possible (according to one prevailing theory of *curanderismo*) because all persons, animals, and certain objects can either emit or absorb vibrating energy (*vibraciones*). This vibrating energy can either be positive or negative in both form and effect. It can cause happiness or sadness, good or evil, good luck or bad luck. The *curandero*, recognizing the supernatural powers and properties of certain material objects, can use these same objects in conjunction with various incantations to alter or correct the vibrating energy surrounding a person. According to this theoretical premise, illness can be considered as a concentration of negative forces within a person's body. These negative forces, depending on their origin and their purpose, can affect a person physically, mentally, or socially. In their efforts to restore their patients' health, the *curanderos* use material objects to manipulate these vibrations, thus altering or correcting the patient's surrounding force field.

The second level of healing, less common than the first, is the spiritual level. In order to work on the spiritual level the *curandero* must enter a trance. *Curanderos* who can work on this level are thought to be able to project their own souls or spirits out of their bodies, making the body a vessel for other spirits. These persons are called mediums. Benevolent spirits then enter the medium's body and take it over, using it to communicate with the patient. The medium is thought to act only as a link between the material and spiritual realms of existence; therefore, the *curanderos* state that it is not the mediums themselves but rather the spirits who do the actual curing. The *curandero* working on this level merely allows his body to be a channel of communication between the spiritual and the material world.

On the spiritual level, illness can be caused, diagnosed, and cured by spiritual forces called *corrientes espirituales* (spiritual currents). The spiritual plane is thought to be a level of existence touching ours, but contact with it can be made only in special circumstances or through special individuals such as mediums, and through the manipulation of spiritual currents. On this level the *curanderos* also deal with patients' problems that can be classified as physical, social, or psychological. The healers manipulate spiritual currents or the spirits themselves.

Work on the mental level is the rarest type of supernatural manipulation. Only a few of the *curanderos* interviewed acknowledged being able to work on the *nivel mental*. The *curanderos* say that this sort of healer works by learning to channel mental energy (*vibraciones mentales*) directly from his mind to the afflicted part of the patient. This energy is thought to work (mind over matter) by directly modifying the afflicted cells in the patient's body through retarding the spread of damaged cells and speeding the growth and healing of healthy areas. This level of healing has so far proven difficult to document, and we have consequently given it less emphasis than it rightfully deserves. As with the other two types of healing, problems of a social, a psychological, and a physical nature could be alleviated by using the techniques available to practitioners who had the gift (*don*) to work on the mental level.

Supernatural illness can manifest itself in any form that the perpetrator (the *brujo* or *espiritu malo* causing the illness) desires. Since health is often defined as a harmonious balance between a person's physical, psychological, and spiritual existence, a supernatural illness can manifest itself as any disruption in a person's integral harmony. If a physical disruption occurs, then a person may have headaches, stomach problems, or an illness that takes the form of something which may be diagnosed as cancer or diabetes. The *curanderos* explained that many cases appear to be a common or natural form of an illness when they actually have a supernatural cause. These diseases can only be cured by supernatural means. Some *curanderos* expressed the concern that people who use only the conventional health-care system are dying needlessly, because the doctors cannot protect them from these supernatural influences—especially since the doctors do not believe in those influences. Once harmed, such patients have no idea where to go for help, since the conventional system will inevitably fail them.

Among the social problems brought about by supernatural forces are bad luck, loss of job, car problems, marital disruptions, drinking problems, and rebellious children. Patients realize that any family is bound to have a certain share of misfortune, but when the misfortune is prolonged and when it takes on a whole series of manifestations rather than appearing to be a single problem, people begin to suspect some extraneous intervention in their lives. If some outside supernatural cause is diagnosed for these accumulated special problems, then the *curandero* becomes active in removing the cause through supernatural means.

In the psychological realm, supernaturally induced illness can appear as common psychological disorders such as nervous breakdowns, paranoia, depression, or excessive worries. Some *curanderos* recognize these states of mind in a classic psychological sense and also recognize the mimicking ones caused by supernatural harm. One of these healers said that many patients placed in mental hospitals are afflicted with psychological problems produced by supernatural illness and are capable of being helped. But, he went on to say, the people treating these patients do not recognize the validity of supernatural disorders and have never consulted anyone capable of helping to solve such problems. He and other *curanderos* believe that if someone could undo the supernatural harm being done to these mental patients, the patients would be capable of leading normal lives and could be immediately discharged.

Since many of the problems that *curanderos* must solve involve manipulations of the supernatural, in essence the *curandero* is dealing with powers beyond scientific recognition or evaluation. *Curanderos* attribute some illnesses to an agent whose existence must be taken on faith. They manipulate objects and employ rituals which supposedly channel and rearrange forces that are currently and perhaps permanently beyond our ability to demonstrate in acceptable scientific paradigms. Therefore, for all practical purposes *curanderismo* deals with magic as opposed to science. However, it must be emphasized that the *curandero*'s magic is not the innocent magic of Walt Disney's Cinderella or Peter Pan, nor is it the distorted and violent magic of Hollywood horror films. The *curandero*'s magic is the far more ancient form of supernatural knowledge found in medieval Europe and dating back to Egypt, India, and pre-Christian Europe. In order to understand this magic it is necessary to put the anthropological study of magic in historical perspective.

Because of its universal presence in cultural systems, magic has been the focus of serious study in anthropology for nearly a century. It was first approached in a systematic fashion by James G. Frazer in a twelve-volume set entitled *The Golden Bough* (Frazer 1922). In that work Frazer set the framework for most existing scientific theories and studies of magic when he described what he called the "Law of Similarity." Within this general law he outlined two principles which form the foundation for social-science analysis of magic: "first, that like produced like, or that effect resembles its cause, and second, that things which have once been in contact with each other continue to act on one another at a distance after the physical contact has been severed" (Frazer 1922:415). Frazer's articulation of these two principles has led to the classification of various magical rites in cultures around the world according to whether they were examples of imitative magic (the first principle) or contagious magic (the second principle).

Equally important to Frazer's articulation of the principles of imitative magic is his definition of the way in which supernatural events occur. He says, "Things act on each other at a distance through a secret sympathy, the impulse being transmitted from one to the other by means of what we might conceive of as an invisible ether . . . to explain how things can physically affect each other through a space which appears to be empty" (Frazer 1922:413). Frazer's formulation of the principles of contact (contagion) and imitation are not at all incompatible with the views of the *curanderos*, at least as their theories pertain to the material level of *curanderismo*.

Many social-science studies of magic have noted the similarity between magical rituals or spells and scientific procedures or formulas. In some cultural systems, Western cultures for example, magic and science even have the same historical roots but somewhat divergent histories. It is often either stated or implied that science turned toward dealing with empirical phenomena while magic remained stagnated by focusing its attention on the supernatural realm. This attitude is significantly different from the view of magic held by *curanderos*. They say that magic is empirical. It deals with objects and observable events; it is based upon a systematic body of knowledge; it has evolved, improved through time by the addition of new knowledge; and it produces results that can be both directly and indirectly perceived, recorded, and tested.

These two views are probably irreconcilable in the minds and behavior of those who maintain one of these perspectives over the other. However, these differences do not need to lead to practical problems in delivering health care to someone who holds one viewpoint or the other. A pragmatic viewpoint exists to deal with this situation. The pragmatic perspective of these conflicting views states that the magic of *curanderismo* is real magic as opposed to fictional or entertainment magic but that it is real in a social sense rather than in the sense of some ultimate scientific reality. It is real because people believe in this magic and believe that it works. They do things, say things, and think things that they would not do, say, or think if they did not believe in magic. Thus, people behave as if magic were real. Since it is this behavior and belief that affects the way people will interact with the scientific medical system, the important point to focus on is not the ultimate reality of magic but the more immediate reality of the patient's perceptions and behavior.

The problem is that this simple pragmatism allows magic to exist without any attempt to explain it or to explain its continued persistence in the face of scientific empiricism. There are plenty of people today who are scientists, in the strictest sense of the word, and also believe in magic and the supernatural. Therefore social scientists have formulated explanations for magic, such as the one proposed by Lucy Mair: "Nobody is willing to resign himself to a sickness with no remedy. The sick person and his family need to feel that something is being done. This may be a matter of finding simple remedies, and these may or may not be effective. But there must be somewhere a theory of causation which can account for the serious cases" (Mair 1969 : 10). Mair goes on to suggest that magic becomes a major theory to explain the causes of illness and misfortune found in societies around the world.

Bronislaw Malinowski (1935, 1948), on the other hand, proposes that magic exists for psychological reasons. He notes that most magic is concentrated in areas where the results of human endeavor are not easily predictable or where there is some doubt about the outcome of a particular event (note the number of superstitious beliefs among athletes and entertainers). He felt that these situations produced acute psychological discomfort for the people involved in them, so they invented magic, which gave them the comforting feeling of being able to control the uncontrollable at least part of the time.

Beatrice Blyth White (1950) suggests that the persistence of magic and sorcery can be explained at least in part by its function as a mechanism to promote social control. This works, according to White, because if a group of people believe in magic, they believe that those who behave badly towards others will be the targets of supernaturally induced harm (sickness, misfortune, and the like). They will therefore be much less likely to get out of control.

E. E. Evans-Pritchard (1937) provides still another explanation for magic in society. He felt that among the Azande, a group of people he worked with in Africa, witchcraft and magic were used to explain unusual, unfortunate, and otherwise inexplicable events. Evans-Pritchard felt that the Azande derived psychological satisfaction from explaining these unfortunate circumstances as magical and that they also derived social satisfaction from the explanation, since it allowed them to retaliate against those they thought were doing the harm. Evans-Pritchard goes on to suggest that similar mechanisms might be operating in other cultures.

Another social-science explanation of magic, at least healing magic, is subscribed to by the present authors. It revolves around the idea that illness within the scientific perspective is impersonal. It affects individuals, but it is caused by impersonal agents, such as a virus, stress, trauma, or social conditions. The scientific framework explains why any individual with a given physical makeup will be affected by a particular environmental condition, but these are impersonal forces affecting everyone equally and do not answer the important question why a particular individual got sick.

Belief in magic personalizes misfortune. The magical theories of disease not only explain what causes an illness but also help explain why the illness struck one person and not another. It provides the victim with a moral, social, or personal explanation of his misfortune, since the disease is viewed as being caused by a recognizable person or force, not an impersonal one.

Magic can also provide the patient with hope when the scientific prognosis is hopeless. For example, from the scientific point of view there is only one conclusion to terminal cancer: death. Acceptance of the diagnosis (and its underlying theory of medicine) means acceptance of that conclusion to the illness. From the magical perspective, no illness that has been caused by magic is incurable. If magic brought about illness or misfortunes, more powerful magic, properly done, can eliminate it. This is one of the basic premises of magic: what can be done can also be undone. The patient's position is hopeless only if he comes to believe that his treatment started too late to help or if the magician countering the magic used against him has less power than the person or entity causing it. In both cases it is likely that the patient would seek help from yet another source, one that he or she felt would bring about a successful cure and a resurgence of hope. At least in the case of chronic or terminal illness, this psychological byproduct of magic—the continuation of hope and expectations for a cure—may explain part of its persistence.

Another reason for the persistence of people's belief in magic is the theoretical paradigm of magic. Both magic and science are based upon a belief in the existence of compulsive formulas. These compulsive formulas describe a constant relationship between cause and effect and can be discovered by the scientist or the magician. A compulsive formula is one which states that if you add A and B together in the proper environment and in the correct sequence, they will produce C. They will always act in this way; they will never produce D, always C. Thus the result is compelled by the nature of the process itself. Science can be seen simply as a process for discovering all of the compulsive formulas that govern the physical universe. Magic is a process for discovering the compulsive formulas that govern the supernatural realm. The corollary to this belief in compulsive formulas is the understanding that if A and B are added together and do not produce C, then the manipulator did something wrong. Compulsive formulas *always* work as long as you use the correct sequence and have the proper environment. Many students have found out that compulsive formulas always work but that a young scientist does not always work them correctly when she is in a freshman chemistry lab trying to make an experiment turn out the way her lab book says it should. But the failure of a would-be scientist does not shake anyone's belief in the validity of science or its compulsive formulas. The failure of a *curandero*, by the same token, does not shake any believer's faith in magic or its compulsive formulas. The client simply considers that particular magician incompetent or unable to perform a certain magical manipulation.

None of these explanations takes into account the *curanderos'* perception of magic. The social scientists are attempting to explain what magic does to or does for a particular group of people as a whole, but they are basing their viewpoint on the belief that magic is probably not real except in a social sense. The *curanderos* believe that magic is real in and of itself and that they can manipulate the supernatural world through their knowledge of magic. The *curanderos* also know that modern medical practitioners do not, as a rule, believe in magic. They even go so far as to fault them for their disbelief. One informant explained that some proportion of all illness is caused by what we would label magic. In mental institutions the number of patients who are magically afflicted may run as high as 10 percent of the total population. According to our informant, these people cannot be cured by conventional means, only by magical ones, so they never get well. Many with physical ailments even die. When we asked the informant how to identify patients who could be helped by magic, he replied that the best way was to have someone like himself screen them. But another way is to look for those mental patients who have the following characteristics: their environment is generally positive; they want help; and others around them are willing to help. In fact, everything is so promising that the therapist often believes that helping such a sufferer will be easy. He is then surprised to find that whatever he tries fails for no apparent reason. Our informant feels that the medical practitioner should re-examine such patients, using magical techniques to look for magical causes of their illness.

Professional *curanderos* generally concentrate on handling serious physical ailments (diabetes, asthma, terminal cancer), on resolving difficult social problems (marital conflicts, family disruptions, business partnerships), on alleviating psychological disturbances (depression, impotency, conversion hysteria), on changing people's fortunes (luck in love, business, or home life) and on removing or guarding against misfortune or illness caused by hexes (*mal puestos*) placed on their patients by a sorcerer (*brujo*) or an evil spirit at the instigation of a rival or enemy. A number of different types of professional *curanderos* exist, and they are distinguished from one another and among themselves primarily by their curing technique or combination of techniques. It is these healers who know about and utilize the theories, as well as the specific practices, of the three technical areas or levels of healing: the material, spiritual, and mental.

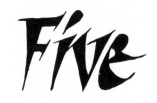

THE
MATERIAL
LEVEL

CURANDERISMO'S THREE LEVELS OF TREATMENT, the material, the spiritual, and the mental, are not mutually exclusive in the treatment of illness or other problems, and most *curanderos* employ combinations which they believe necessary to benefit their patients. The material level is the easiest of the three to describe; it is the most extensively practiced and the most widely reported. At this level, the *curandero* manipulates physical objects and performs rituals which create an atmosphere conducive to treatment. Ritual behavior alters the client's awareness of his or her problems, and the treatment procedure relieves pain, anxiety, depression, insecurity, or whatever ails the patient. Combinations of objects and rituals (sometimes called spells or works, *trabajos*) are widely recognized by Mexican Americans as having curative powers. However, the power and significance of the objects and rituals are not widely understood, and this allows room for unscrupulous practices and can lead to misunderstandings about *curanderos* on the part of the public.

Perhaps the outstanding characteristic of the objects used at the material level is that they are common items used for everyday activities such as cooking. Practitioners at the material level employ herbs such as *oregano*, *manzanilla*, and *anis*; fruits (oranges, lemons, and papaya); nuts such as pecans; flowers (roses and geraniums); animals and animal products (chickens, doves, and eggs); and spices (onions, garlic, and black pepper). Religious symbols are also widely used (for example, the crucifix, pictures of saints, incense, candles, holy water, oils, and sweet fragrances). Secular items like cards, alum, and ribbons are used. The *curandero* makes his patients rely extensively on their own resources by prescribing items that either are familiar or have strong cultural significance.

Medicinal herbs are much employed by *curanderos* at the material level. These herbs are usually prescribed as teas, herbal baths, or poultices. The teas can be considered a sort of primitive chemotherapy. *Borraja*, for example, is taken to cut a fever; *flor de tila*, a mild sedative, is taken for insomnia; *yerba de la golondrina* is used as a douche for vaginal discharges; and *estilos de helote* are used for kidney problems. Herbal baths are usually prescribed to deal with skin diseases; for example, *fresno* is used to treat scalp problems such as eczema, dandruff, and psoriasis, and *linaza* is prescribed for sores that appear all over the body. For specific sores like boils, *malva* leaves, for example, are boiled until soft and then applied to the sore as a poultice. Another function of herbs is their use as decongestants. A handful of oregano is placed in a humidifier to promote breathing in persons with a bad cold. If anything distinguishes Mexican American *curanderos* from other folk healers, it is their knowledge and use of a wide variety of medicinal herbs.

A few of the more traditional *curanderos* classify herbs as having the dichotomous properties (hot/cold and wet/dry) considered essential for humoral medicine. Using these dual properties, any given herb or combination of herbs may be prescribed, depending on the characteristics of the illness. If an illness is supposedly caused by excessive heat, an herb with cold properties is given. Conversely, if an illness is believed to be caused by excessive coldness and dryness, a combination of herbs having hot and wet properties is given.

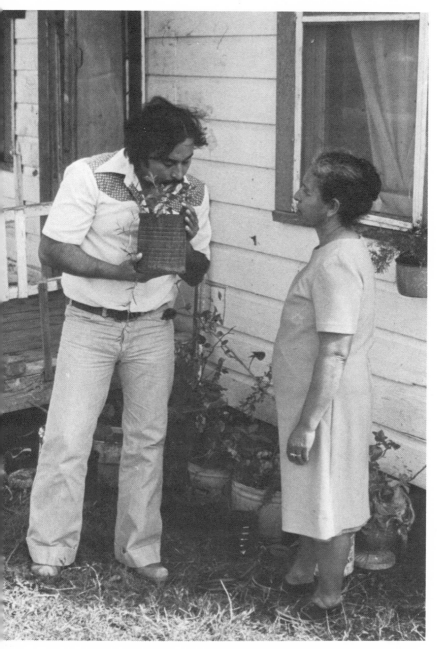

Curandera instructing an apprentice in the use of herbal remedies

In south Texas, this humoral concept of medicine is not very prevalent among the general population; however, some *curanderos* still depend on this theory to classify illnesses and to prescribe herbal treatment.

Many *curanderos* recognize herbs for their chemical properties—poisons (*yerba del coyote*), hallucinogens (*peyote*), sedatives (*flor de tila*), stimulants (*yerba del trueno*), and purgatives (*cascara sagrada*). Most of these healers do not refer to the hot/cold classification of illness; rather, they indicate the beneficial chemical properties of the herbs that allow them to cure natural illnesses.

Some herbs are also used for their spiritual properties. Spiritual cleansings (*barridas*) are often given with *ruda*, *romero*, and *albacar*. Herbs are also used as amulets. For example, *verbena*, worn as an amulet, is used to help open a person's mind so that he or she may be better able to learn and retain knowledge.

Not all herbal lore is passed on as an oral tradition. Books from Mexico which give a sophisticated description and classification of herbs are now being widely circulated among *curanderos*. One such book (Capo n.d.) describes *borraja* (borage) as a diuretic and as able to promote sweating. It says that the herb acts directly on the kidneys and increases the quantity of urine. The properties of *borraja* include cutting a fever, and it is thought to improve the circulation of the blood. Tea made from *borraja* is said to be helpful for the evolution of fever-based eruptions such as measles and scarlet fever. Its ability to promote sweating helps prevent complications. It also aids recovery in illnesses of the breathing tract such as bronchitis caused by flu or pneumonia. Its diuretic action also favors the elimination of toxins from the body. The book directs that the tea be made from the flowers and leaves of the *borraja* plant.

But even though these books are readily accessible, many people still rely on the *curanderos* for advice on what herbs to use, because books often ignore a very important problem of the treatment procedure: establishing the correct dosage. How much of the herb should be used in a given amount of water? How many times a day is the tea drunk, and when, and for how many days? Incidentally, these important pieces of information are also sometimes missing from scientific descriptions of the use of medicinal herbs.

The ritual preparation of herbal remedies is also often overlooked in the available catalogues of herbal compounds. Some informants indicated that these *remedios* work if they are simply applied mechanically, but that they work much better if certain precautions are taken in preparing the herbs. There is a series of preparation rites that should be followed. The healer should ask the plant for permission to cut its branches and inform it of the reason why these branches are needed. This rite establishes a spiritual bond between the healer, the plant, and the patient, and it enhances the healing process. It is said that healers who do not comply with these preparation rites are involved in rote behavior and fail to satisfy the proper procedures of the healing process, thereby making their treatments less successful.

Herbs are so important in Mexican American folk medicine that the use of herbs is often confused with the art of *curanderismo* itself. Indeed, *curanderismo* depends on the use of herbs to such an extent that some *curanderos* specialize in herbs. These *curanderos* are usually known as *yerberos* or *yerberas*. But their knowledge and skill goes beyond the mere formula: one disease, one herbal treatment. In order for a *curandero* to be genuine, even at the material level, an element of mysticism must be involved. And some *curanderos* have successful practices without ever making use of herbs.

Because of the strong orientation toward spiritual and supernatural forces in Mexican American folk medicine, religious symbols are very evident in *curanderismo*. Special invocations are commonly directed at saints or spirits to bring about special results. For example, San Martin de Porres is asked to relieve poverty, San Martin Caballero to help in business, San Judas Tadeo to help in impossible situations, and Santa Marta to bring harmony to a household. Besides officially recognized saints, *curanderos* also call on spirits who may be considered folk saints—spiritual beings believed to have miraculous powers and given popular respect and veneration without official sanction from the Church (see Romano 1965). Recognized folk saints such as Don Pedrito Jaramillo and El Niño Fidencio are called upon to help the *curandero* in both difficult and routine situations. Other benevolent spirits, such as Allan Kardec, the founder of the spiritualist movement, or relatives and friends of either the *curandero* or the patient, may also be called upon for help.

Water and fire (candles) are sacred objects that allow the *curandero* to control and channel the supernatural powers he has at his disposal. Water, especially holy water, represents a physical link with the spiritual world. Whenever a *curandero* is undertaking a difficult cure, he surrounds himself and his patient with a ring of water to keep away negative influences. Specially prepared water (*agua preparada*) can be rubbed on a person's forehead and cerebellum for strength and protection in healing and spiritual sessions. Other objects such as eggs, lemons, and herbs can also be dipped into this prepared water to enhance their curative powers. Don Pedrito Jaramillo, perhaps the best-known and one of the more successful *curanderos* in south Texas and northern Mexico, prescribed water in almost all his treatments (see Hudson 1951; Romano 1964).

Fire is used to establish direct communication with the supernatural. Fire, or a flame, represents the presence of a supernatural order which can help create or destroy all types of influences affecting a human being. Flickering candlelight can repel unwanted spiritual beings (*espiritus obscuros*) and attract benevolent spirits (*espiritus de luz*). The use of fire by *curanderos* is analogous to the use of fire in Catholic rituals (candles and incense). Whenever a person wishes to ask a special favor or special protection from the Virgin or a saint, he lights a candle and says a prayer. Fire in the form of a candle establishes a link between the suppliant and the benevolent supernatural spirit who has the power to grant a favor.

Fire is also used as a purifier. Fire is an essential element in most of the termination rites of a healing session. The tools used in a healing session, with the obvious exception of water, are frequently burned to destroy the negative vibrations which have contaminated these objects. These burning rites literally destroy the causes of the illness which was afflicting the patient.

Perfumes, oils, and incense are used by *curanderos* to attract benevolent spirits whenever someone needs special favors or protection. All these objects emit fragrances and vibrations which are pleasing to the spiritual world, making them essential objects in all rituals. In a general sense, oils are used for protection against some perceived harm. *Aceite de vibora* (rattlesnake oil) is said to stop a person from gossiping, and *aceite de las siete potencias* is used to remove bad luck and bad intentions wished on a person. Perfume is used to attract desired outcomes. Perfumes and oils are prescribed for persons who have problems attracting the opposite sex or obtaining a job. Incense is used to bring harmony to a social environment (peace to a household or success to a business establishment, for instance).

At the psychological level, some *curanderos* feel that these particular objects have a strong self-suggestive power, since the patient can see that something is being done to help him. One *curandero* said that in some cases these objects are used only for the patient's sake, not because they are useful in themselves. The patient expects to see something being done, and the *curandero* obliges by lighting candles or burning incense even though these activities are not necessary for a cure.

Lemons, garlic, and purple onions are some of the vegetable objects used by *curanderos* in their work. These objects are used because they are thought to have an intrinsic supernatural or spiritual power (classified as "mana" by anthropologists) to absorb or destroy negative vibrations and to strengthen positive vibrations. The lemon, for example, can be used to represent a person and absorb all his negative influences, and it can also be used to give strength, or positive influences, to a sick person. The lemon also serves as a source of strength whenever a person is in difficult circumstances. Some *curanderos* recommend squeezing a lemon with the left hand whenever a person is undertaking a difficult business meeting, an examination, a legal encounter, or any other uncertain circumstance.

Purple onions and garlic are used to give the patient protection from harm. These objects are believed to have the power to repel negative influences. The patient is cleansed (swept) with garlic or purple onions for protection; it is a sort of spiritual or psychological inoculation. The patient can then return to his environment with some assurance of protection, even if someone wants to harm him.

The animal object most commonly used by south Texas *curanderos* is the egg, although black chickens and doves are also used. In *curanderismo*, some ritual treatments, especially those dealing with supernatural illness, demand that a sacrificial object be used, and the egg qualifies as an animal cell. These objects are believed to have the power to absorb the negative influences or harm (sickness) being done to the patient. After the ritual these objects, and the harm they have absorbed, are usually destroyed by fire, and the patient recovers.

According to Turner (1969 : 19) a ritual is "prescribed formal behavior for occasions not given over to technological routine, having reference to beliefs in mystical beings or powers." Many rituals involve the manipulation of physical objects together with prayers or invocations, and thus they are common at the material level of *curanderismo*.

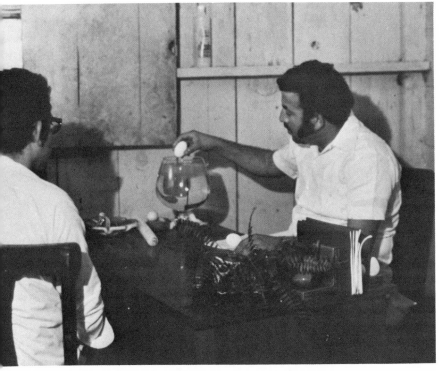

Curandero preparing an egg to be used in a cure *(Photograph by Aida Hurtado)*

The basic ritual at the material level is the *barrida* or spiritual cleansing. The purpose of these cleansings is to eliminate the negative forces or vibrations influencing a patient by transferring them to another object. This is classified as transference magic. A second purpose is to give the patient spiritual strength and thereby enhance his recovery. The objects most commonly used in *barridas* are eggs, lemons, garlic, purple onions, doves, and black chickens, along with *piedra alumbre* (alum), candles, oils, perfumes, incense, and the stalks or branches of certain herbs such as *albacar, ruda* and *romero*.

A *barrida* literally means "a sweeping." While being swept, the client may either be standing or lying down and

must be concentrating on his Maker, or any other benevolent influence or spirit. Some *curanderos* perform the
sweeping ritual while the patient is sitting, but we are told
by some *curanderos* that this is not the correct procedure.

Patients are swept from their head to their feet, with the
curandero making sweeping or brushing motions with an
egg, a lemon, an herb, or whatever appropriate object is
deemed necessary. According to some informants the object
must be held in the *curandero*'s left hand and must touch
the person being swept. The person is swept in front, in
back, and on the sides. If a particular part of the body is in
pain special attention is given to the affected area. While
sweeping the patient, the *curandero* usually recites specific
prayers that appeal to God, saints, or other spiritual beings
to restore health to the patient. The *curandero* may recite
these prayers out loud or silently. In either case, the presence of the *curandero*, the soothing effect of the sweepings (touching), and the low-keyed monotone chant of the
prayers produce in the patient a light trance state that is
comforting and reassuring. Standard prayers used in this ritual include the Lord's Prayer, the Apostles' Creed, and *Las
doce verdades del mundo* ("The Twelve Truths of the
World"; see appendix).

Turner (1967:27–35) identifies three properties of a ritual symbol. One is condensation, which means that many
things and actions are represented by one symbol. Another
is unification, which means that disparate significances "are
interconnected by virtue of their common possession of
analogous qualities or by association in fact or thought." For
example, what does a lemon or an egg have to do with
health? The third property, polarization, has to do with the
mystical and material properties of the ritual symbol. The
material properties of the egg include its ordinary use as
food; its mystical properties, however, include its ability to
absorb negative influences (sickness) from a patient. The following description of a *barrida* given by one of our infor-

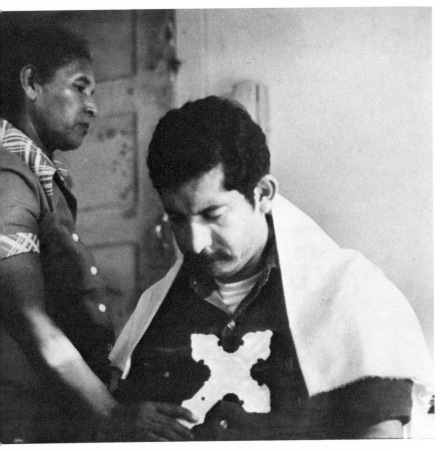

Patient being given a *barrida* with a crucifix

mants illustrates how the material objects, the mystical power of these objects, the invocations, the *curandero*, and the patient come together and form a healing ritual:

This was a case in which the condition or illness was provoked. In other words, using these means [*curanderismo*] persons can be either helped or harmed; that is, persons who are healthy can become ill with any given illness. This is what people call *mal puesto* [provoked harm].

In this case five eggs, four lemons, some branches of *albacar* [sweet basil] and oil will be used. In some cases it is necessary to use animals to execute the cure. These animals would have to be sacrificed, but in this case the eggs come to represent the living animals, being in themselves living cells which will give the formation of an animal. The use of the lemons is due to the fact that they are often used to harm persons as well as being used to cure them. Lemons possess certain power within the conjuring and enchantment procedures of the occult sciences.

To begin the healing process the lemons and eggs are washed with alcohol or water; it is desirable that they be clean [ritually purified] in order to execute the healing ritual. Before beginning the ritual, the participants must take off their rings, watches, and other jewelry. Once the healing process begins, high-frequency spiritual and mental vibrations come into effect, which can produce electrical discharges on the metal, causing disturbances which can disrupt the healing process.

The sweeping itself is done by interchanging an egg and a lemon successively until the ritual is completed. Sweeping with the egg is intended to transfer the problem from the patient to the egg by means of conjures and invocations. The lemon is used to dominate the *trabajo* which has been placed on the patient, thereby facilitating the healing process.

The patient is also swept once with *albacar* which has been rinsed in *agua preparada* [specially prepared water]. This sweeping serves as a purification for the patient, intended to give strength and comfort to his spiritual being. The ritual ends by making crosses with *aceite pre-*

parado [specially prepared oil] on the principal joints of the patient, e.g. neck, under the knees, and above the elbow. This oil is especially prepared and serves to cut the negative currents and vibrations which surround the patient, which have been placed there by whoever is provoking the harm. The crosses also serve as protection against the continued effect of these negative vibrations. *Agua preparada* is then rubbed on the patient's forehead and cerebellum [*cerebro*] to tranquilize him and to give him mental strength.

All the objects used in the *barrida* are then burned in order to destroy the negative influences or harm which has been transferred from the patient.

This informant refused to reveal the prayers he uses in his healing rituals. He says that he usually works alone and does not want his enemies to find out his special and private invocations. He does explain that both water and oil are prepared with mental vibrations, which give these objects *propiedades magneticas* (magnetic properties). These properties give strength to whatever objects come in contact with the water or with the oil.

Another ritual is the *sahumerio* or incensing. The *sahumerio* is strictly a purification rite and is used for treating businesses, households, farms, and sometimes patients. This ritual is executed by first preparing hot coals, then placing an appropriate incense on the coals. The *curandero* may prepare his own incense, or he may prescribe some commercial incense which is already prepared, such as *el sahumerio maravilloso* (marvelous or miraculous incense). Every room or living space in the house is incensed thoroughly by carrying a pan with the smoking incense through the building, making sure that all corners, closets, and hidden spaces, such as under the beds, are properly incensed (filled with smoke). While the healer is incensing a house, he or someone else reads or recites an appropriate prayer. If the *sahumerio maravilloso* is used, the prayer is to Santa Marta, asking that peace and harmony be restored to the household. After the *sahumerio*, the healer may sprinkle holy water on the floor of every room in the house and then light a white candle which stays lit for seven days.

The *sahumerio* is an instance where the *curandero* treats the social environment while seeking to bring about a change in the lifestyle and living conditions of the persons who live or work there. Incensing of a house is thought to do away with negative influences such as bad luck (*salaciones*), marital disruptions, illness, or disharmony. For businesses and farms, incensing helps assure success and growth and gives protection against jealous competitors.

Another type of ritual, called a *sortilegio* (conjure), may use material objects like ribbons to tie up the negative influences that harm the *curandero*'s patients. These negative influences are frequently personal shortcomings such as excessive drinking, infidelity, rebellious children, unemployment, or any other problem believed to be imposed by antisocial magic (*un trabajo*). One *sortilegio* that we observed required four ribbons: one red, one green, one white, and one black, each about one yard in length. Each ribbon stands for a type of magic (red, green, white, and black magic) which may have been used to affect the client. The four ribbons, one on top of the other, are placed on the floor in a straight line. The petitioner is then asked to walk over them, forward and backward, three times. While walking over the ribbons, the petitioner and the healer say an invocation (*conjuro y rechazo*) rejecting all malevolent forces which may be intended for the petitioner:

En el nombre de la Santisima Trinidad, Dios Padre,
Dios Hijo y Dios Espiritu Santo, conjuro y rechazo los
trabajos rojos, los trabajos negros; los conjuro a los siete
mares rojos, a los siete mares negros. En el nombre de

*Dios conjuro y rechazo todo el mal que me haigan
hecho. Conjuro a mis enemigos carnados o desencarnados. En el nombre de Dios aqui encierro a mis enemigos
y mis enemigas.*

In the name of the Holy Trinity, God the Father, God the
Son, and God the Holy Spirit, I conjure and I reject the
red works, the black works; I conjure them to the seven
red seas, the seven black seas. In the name of God, I conjure and reject all the evil that has been done to me. I
conjure my enemies in the flesh and without the flesh.
In the name of God I lock up my enemies here.

The petitioner continues the invocation by knotting all four
ribbons at the same time. While knotting, the petitioner and
the healer invoke the following conjure:

*En el nombre de Dios, aqui encierro mis enemigos y mis
enemigas. Pido mi felicidad y buena suerte, salud y di-
nero. Por todos los seres dominadores, que se vayan
todos los maleficios a los siete mares rojos y a los siete
mares negros. Por todos los seres dominadores, aqui encierro a mis enemigos, aqui los ato y los conjuro a todos
mis enemigos carnados y desencarnados, en el nombre
de Dios todopoderoso.*

In the name of God, here I lock up my enemies. I ask for
my happiness, good luck, health and money. By all the
dominating spirits, may the evil doings depart to the
seven red seas and the seven black seas. By all the dominating beings, I here lock up my enemies. I here tie and
conjure all my enemies in the flesh and without the
flesh. In the name of all powerful God.

The completely knotted ribbons are placed in an empty
jar, and the petitioner is instructed to repeat the following
invocation while screwing the lid down tight:

Ahora aqui encierro a mis enemigos y mis enemigas, y que me dejen en paz.

Now I here lock my enemies, and they will leave me in peace.

The jar is buried or hidden in a safe place, and so are the petitioner's problems.

A ritual intended to influence people from a distance is the act of candle burning (*velaciones*). There are two main symbols in candling, color and the position of the candle or the configuration of multiple candles. Blue candles are burned for serenity or tranquility. Red candles are burned for health, power, or domination. Pink candles are burned for good will. Green candles are burned to remove a harm or a negative influence, and purple candles are burned to repel and attack bad spirits (*espiritus obscuros*). If a petitioner asks for protection, the candles may be burned in a triangle. The triangle is considered to be the strongest formation, one whose influence cannot be broken easily. If the petitioner wants to dominate someone—a spouse, a lover, an adversary—the candles may be burned in circles. Other formations include crosses, rectangles, and squares (see Buckland 1970), depending on the results desired.

Candles have other uses than as direct spells. A diagnosis can be made by studying the flame of the candle, the ridges, and figures which appear on the melted wax. For example, a patient may be swept with a candle, the healer reciting an invocation asking the spirit of the patient to allow its material being to be investigated for any problems, physical or spiritual, which may be affecting him. Lighting the candle after the *barrida* will aid the *curandero* to reveal the patient's problems. Similarly, if a petitioner asks for a candling, the wax of the burned candles may be examined for figures or other messages which point to the source of a patient's problems.

The preceding list of material objects, rituals, and prayers is by no means exhaustive. Its purpose is to give an indication of how, at the material level, a *curandero* combines material objects, prayers, and invocations in healing rituals which address themselves to physical, social, and psychological problems. Since the concern here is to describe healing procedures, the rituals and objects used by those who manipulate negative forces to harm people (*brujos*) are not included. However, it must be emphasized that harming rituals do exist, and that they are used.

The material level is more widely known and more widely reported than either the spiritual or the mental level because many of its procedures can be reduced to simple healing formulas. The so-called Mexican American folk illnesses (*mal ojo, empacho*, and *susto*, for example) so widely discussed in the literature, are treated at the material level. However, taking the rituals at their face value has caused some confusion or lack of appreciation of the ritual procedures involved with these illnesses. This happens because the healers' theoretical assumptions are often left out of scholarly discussions or analyses. Left out as well is any discussion of the mystical meaning of the ritual's symbols. We have tried to weave these omissions into the following examples of healing that were given to us by our informants.

Most of these healing formulas were contributed by an informant who has been a practicing *curandera* for over twenty years. She began healing as a young girl treating only members of her family, and it was not until after she got married that she was convinced to develop her potential as a healer. Her list of healing formulas represents types of illnesses with which this informant and other *curanderos* deal, organized according to her theoretical perspective. These illnesses may range from the simple to the very complex, from the so-called Mexican American folk illnesses to apparently serious psychological problems. In her long practice our informant has dealt with many problems and many situations, and the following list in no way does justice to her skill or her knowledge.

Our informant was asked to describe the popular Mexican American folk illnesses, including *susto, mal ojo, caida de mollera, empacho,* and *bilis.* She stated that these illnesses are treated at the material level, using the objects, rituals, and prayers commonly employed by *curanderos.* However, they are not often treated by the *curanderos* themselves. The widespread knowledge of these rituals in Mexican American communities may be the reason why persons who treat these illnesses are often labeled as professional *curanderos* by social scientists. Our informant told us that she and other full-time healers only dealt with the most serious cases of these illnesses, since in most instances they could be and were treated by almost anyone in the community without resorting to a professional *curandero.* Her description of these problems follows:

SUSTO

Susto [fright; sometimes thought of as loss of soul] can affect anyone from a young baby to an elderly person. The more serious illness is called *susto pasado,* a person who has been ill with fright for a long time. A person with *susto pasado* suffers from stomach trouble, diarrhea, lack of appetite, lethargy, irritability, and loss of weight. Persons can be frightened at home, at work, in their sleep, or just about anywhere. Even if a person is brave, his body may be surprised and frightened. *Susto* can sometimes be diagnosed by touching the person's nose; it should be very soft, like cotton.

The cure may be done with an old broom. The sick person lies down and is completely covered with a sheet. The healer [*el que cura*] sweeps the patient with the broom, saying the Apostles' Creed three times. At the end of each Creed, the healer whispers in the patient's ear, "Come, don't stay there" [*Vente no te quedes alli*].

The patient responds, "I am coming" [*Aqui vengo*]. The sick person must perspire and is then given some tea of *yerba anis* to drink. The healer then places a cross of holy palm on the patient's head and asks Almighty God, in the name of the Holy Trinity, to restore the patient's spiritual strength.

CAIDA DE MOLLERA

Caida de mollera [fallen fontanelle] may be caused by pulling the baby's bottle from his mouth while he is sucking, by a fall from the bed or crib, or by throwing the baby up in the air. The symptoms are diarrhea and irritability [as well as a depressed fontanelle].

This illness is treated by wetting the baby's head with warm water and soaping the soft spot really well. The healer then gently places his fingers inside the baby's mouth and pushes up on his palate; with the other hand he gently pulls the hairs on the baby's soft spot. In some cases the healer places warm water in his mouth, and places his mouth on the baby's soft spot, and gently sucks in.

EMPACHO

Empacho is caused by having food stick to the stomach lining. In some cases specific foods which are believed hard to digest, such as popcorn, cause *empacho*. *Empacho* is also caused by forcing a child to eat food he does not like or want. Some mothers give their children too much to eat; this also causes *empacho*.

Empacho can be treated by giving the child a purgative. In order to treat the "damaged stomach" a tea is also given such as *te de rosa de castilla* or *te de yerba del gato*. In some cases the healer massages that part of the back behind the stomach with warm olive oil and pulls on the skin. The skin is said to make a snapping noise when the trapped food particles are loosened. In either case, a tea is given to treat the damaged stomach.

MAL OJO

Mal ojo [literally translated "bad eye"] is caused by persons with "strong vision" admiring a child, a grown person, or an object. If these persons fail to touch whoever or whatever they are admiring, their strong vision causes that person to be ill or that object to be damaged. The symptoms in children are usually irritability, fever, headaches, vomiting, and drooping eyes.

Mal ojo is treated by having the child lie down and sweeping him three times with an egg. The sweeping is done by forming crosses (*crusitas*) with the egg, on the child's body, starting at the head and going to the feet. While sweeping, the healer recites the Apostles' Creed three times, making sure that he sweeps both the front and the back. The egg is cracked and dropped into a glass or jar filled with water. The jar may then be placed on the child's head, and another Creed recited. The jar is then placed under the child's bed, usually under the place where the child rests his head. The next morning at sunrise the egg may either be burned or cast away in the form of a cross.

BILIS

Another popular illness sometimes described in the literature is *bilis*, which is excessive bile in a person's system caused by extreme anger or fear. This excessive bile becomes concentrated in the person's stomach or intestines. If the person suffers from *bilis* for long periods of time, the illness may progress to *bilis cuajada* (coagulated bile). *Bilis cuajada* causes inflammation of the stomach or of the intestines. Symptoms of *bilis* include gas, constipation, a dirty white tongue, and a sour, bitter, and dry mouth.

Bilis is treated by taking laxatives once a week for three weeks. Commercial laxatives such as epsom salts

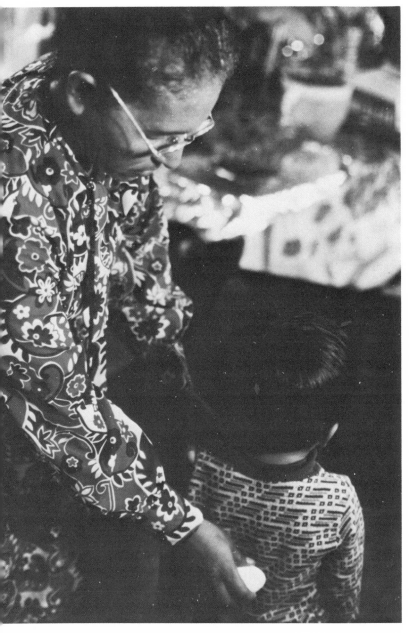

Child being cured of *mal de ojo* with an egg

or purgative herbs such as *cascara sagrada* (sacred bark) are recommended. The idea is to cleanse the stomach of all the accumulated bile and restore it to normal.

Curanderos recognize that some illnesses are brought about by natural causes, such as improper function of the body, carelessness, or the inability of a person to take care of himself. *Curanderos* often talk openly about infectious and contagious diseases. At the material level, natural illnesses are usually treated with herbs. The following are some examples of herbal treatments of natural illnesses:

HEMORRHAGE
The rose [*rosa de castillo*] treats hemorrhages, infections, and sores. Whenever a person has a hemorrhage, place three roses in water, boil them, and make the person drink the tea. The geranium also cures menstruating women of excessive bleeding. A tea is made either of five geranium leaves or one flower. The afflicted person drinks this tea for nine consecutive days, preferably before breakfast.

VAGINAL DISCHARGES
Some vaginal infections are caused in women who do not abstain from intercourse for the required number of days after giving birth. These vaginal infections are yellow or white. These infections are treated by giving the patient a tea made from herbs called *la cachana y el cachano*. The tea is made from two leaves and is taken twice daily, in the morning and in the evening. The person also takes a warm bath made from the following herbs: *yerba anis, yerba buena, ruda, mejorana,* and *yerba de San Nicolas;* these herbs are boiled together. After the bath the person is heavily clothed in order to perspire. The person has to perspire in order for the illness to come out.

GALL STONES

Cactus tea [*te de nopal*] is recommended for gall stones.
The biggest part of the cactus is cut and the pulp removed. This pulp is boiled and the tea is used by the
patient as drinking water. If the stones are too big and an
operation is required, then cactus tea will not help. However, if the stones are not too big and the illness is not
too serious, cactus tea helps to get rid of the stones. Cactus is also good to cure infections.

FEVERS

Fever can be cured by either using herbs or poultices.
Borraja and *huachachile* cure fevers because both have
cold properties. The tea of either plant can be given to
the patient in order to cut his fever. Poultices to cut fever
are also made from raw meat mixed with vinegar and
onions. If meat is not available, then dough can be sub-
stituted. The dough is mixed with vinegar to make the
poultice. This poultice is placed on the patient's forehead, stomach, back, and the soles of his feet. The sick
person has to perspire very much in order for the illness
to come out.

SKIN DISEASES

The *fresno* [ash tree] treats skin infections such as
itches, sores, white spots, or scalings. Branches of the
fresno are boiled in a pail and added to the patient's
bathing water. The patient takes as many baths as necessary to cure the infection. *Fresno* can also be used to
tighten loose skin by persons who lose weight in short
periods of time.

Supernatural illnesses (caused by impelling negative forces)
can sometimes be confused with natural illnesses. The
same informant stated that these supernatural illnesses may
be diagnosed as ulcers, tuberculosis, rheumatism, or migraine headaches, but in reality they are believed to be

daños (harms) placed on the person by an enemy. The difference between a natural and a supernatural illness is that physicians cannot cure a supernatural illness. *Curanderos* say that some patients, after spending time and money consulting physicians, realize that physicians cannot help them. They then turn to the *curandero* for help.

MIGRAINE HEADACHES

Migraine headaches can be given to a person by giving that person certain powders in his food or drink. They can also be caused by burning candles whose purpose is to make that person ill. The afflicted person is swept with an egg, the healer [*el que cura*] usually reciting the Apostles' Creed or the Twelve Truths of the World. The egg is broken and placed in a glass of water to make a diagnosis. If the white of the egg forms points with bubbles, then the person is being harmed by a *velacion* [candle burning]. If the egg also has red spots, then the *velacion* is made of red candles in a circle. If the egg has black spots, the powders are being used to harm the patient. Once the diagnosis is made, the patient is given nine *barridas* [cleansings] for nine consecutive days. The first three *barridas* are all done with an egg, the second three with lemons, and the third three with purple onions. An incision in the form of the cross is made on each purple onion and three peppers are placed in the incision. In all cases the objects are burned in live coals after each *barrida*. During the same nine days, the *curandero* burns a green *velacion* in the form of a triangle. The triangle protects the patient from further harm and destroys the harm already being done. When the candles are lit, an invocation is usually said to a saint or benevolent spirit to aid the candles in restoring the patient back to health.

The patient is prescribed a *cocimiento* [a tea]; this tea is usually made of *ruda* [rue] and *yerba del Cristo* [herb of Christ], which must be taken in the morning before breakfast. If the patient was given something to eat or to drink, the healer recommends a laxative to be taken with *chocolate mexicano* [Mexican hot chocolate].

SORES

Some people develop skin eruptions because of some *trabajo* [work] that has been done on them with oils. These oils may be placed on the person's clothing, their work tools, or wherever it is certain that these oils will be touched by the victims. These people are given a series of baths, usually from seven to twenty-one, made with *fresno* [ash tree], lemon, and *yerba del pajaro* [herb of the swallow]. Some bad skin sores also need *barridas*. The egg for these *barridas* has to be from a black hen. These people may also be given a specially prepared incensing [*sahumerio*] such as the *sahumerio de San Cipriano*. This incensing will cleanse the patients of all evil that has been done to them.

RHEUMATISM OR ARTHRITIS

There are some persons who are unable to use their hands, arms, legs, or feet. A figure is usually made of these people and their limbs are stuck to their bodies with needles. For all practical purposes these people become frozen. Other people get their needles stuck one at a time, so it takes them longer to become paralyzed.

These patients are usually given a series of nine *barridas*, for nine consecutive days. The first three *barridas* are given with lemons, the second three with duck eggs, and the last three with black chickens. These barridas are usually concentrated on the patient's afflicted parts with the healer reciting the "Twelve Truths." Strong invocations are also made to saints and other benevolent spirits to aid in the cure. Invocations may also be made to evil spirits asking them to release the patient and restore him back to health. Some black chickens used in the last three *barridas* die right away or within a few days. In some cases the black chickens are burned immediately after the *barrida* to destroy the harm they have trapped in their bodies. The patient is also anointed with holy oil and rubbed with specially prepared alcohol.

Supernatural influences can also disrupt a person's mental health and living environment. At this level the *curandero* deals with social disruption, personality complexes, and sometimes with what seem to be serious psychological disturbances.

MARRIAGES

Some couples may be having problems in getting married, either because of family problems, inability to find a job, etc. They come and ask for help in solving their problem so they can get married. Some healers read their cards to determine if something or someone is blocking their way to prevent them from getting married. If a negative intention is blocking their marriage plans, the *curandero* may give them a series of *barridas* . . . nine or seven . . . with roses and holy candles. The persons are usually wrapped in a white cloth while they are being cleansed; they are also prescribed baths with roses. The *curandero* also lights a white *velacion* [candle burning] in a circle to conclude the marriage.

HOUSEHOLD PROBLEMS

There are some persons who have all kinds of household problems; they cannot find work, they have no food, there is constant illness [in the family], their car breaks down, they cannot get along with other people. These people usually have had a *salacion* [bad luck] placed on them. This is usually done by spreading some powders or graveyard dust on their house so everything will go wrong. These people usually have to be given nine *barri-*

das with fire on nine consecutive days. The first three barridas are given with branches of three herbs: *albacar, ruda,* and *romero.* The second three *barridas* are given with a wide, dried pepper. The pepper is dried and stuffed with romero, seven teeth of garlic, three cloves, and two cinnamon sticks. After each *barrida,* the objects are burned in live coals. After the sixth *barrida,* the persons are cleansed with a combination of three incenses: *myrrha, estoraque,* and *copal.* The last three *barridas* are given with garlic; this garlic is also burned after each *barrida.* This ritual is supposed to be very powerful because it signifies the power of life; it does away with all evil and protects the household from future harm. The persons may also be prescribed *baños especiales de fortuna* (specially prepared baths of good fortune).

INFERIORITY COMPLEX
Some persons feel that everyone looks down on them, or feel that everyone treats them badly. They are unable to get along with people and have few friends. These people are usually given three *barridas* with different colored roses, an oleander branch, and a *ruda* branch. An invocation is made to benevolent spirits to give this person spiritual strength and to help him find himself. This person is also prescribed seven baths with seven herbs, usually *albacar, ruda, romero, yerba buena, verbena, mejorana,* and *anis.* After the three *barridas,* the person is given a *sahumerio* for good luck. He may also be encouraged to use specially prepared perfumes that will help him get along with others.

When asked if she treated mental illness, the informant gave the following case:

This is a specific mental case—very difficult. This patient worked for the street-maintenance department of a small city in south Texas. Every day after work a voice would lead him out into the brush and sometimes keep him there till 2:00 A.M. This activity was wearing out the man and his family and he was going crazy. A bad spirit was following this man, and would not leave him alone. This man was cured, but it took three people to cure him: myself, a friend, and a master (*maestro*) from Mexico. This man was given three *barridas* each day for seven days, one by each of us. The tools used were eggs, lemons, herbs, garlic, and black chickens. The man was also prescribed herbal baths and some teas to drink. He was also given a charm made from the *haba marina* designed to ward off any more negative influences which might be directed at him. This patient regained his sanity.

The examples just described should give the reader an idea of how the *curandero* uses material resources in order to treat patients. Some rituals are rather elaborate and some are quite simple, but all incorporate the use of material objects. As we have seen, an outstanding characteristic of the material level is the *curandero*'s ability to manipulate symbols which are recognized as very much a part of the patient's culture. This *curandera* shares with her patients a common view of the world: she understands their problems and the source of their problems, she is familiar with their lifestyles, and she shares some of their health beliefs and practices. Moreover, the patient's family is asked to participate in most cases. The family helps to locate objects needed (for example, herbs, candles, lemons), participates in the healing rituals by being present and by joining in prayer, and becomes instrumental in getting the patient to follow the *curandera*'s instructions. This combination of ease of communication and ample involvement with the patient and his family gives the *curandera* the advantage of having not only all the information needed for therapeutic purposes but also the reinforced cooperation of the patient and some control over the patient's following through with his treatment procedures. In essence, the *curandera* gathers information, manipulates symbols, prescribes, and involves the patient's total social system in the healing process.

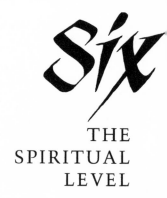

THE
SPIRITUAL
LEVEL

CURANDEROS WHO HAVE THE GIFT (*el don*) for working on the spiritual level (*nivel espiritual*) of *curanderismo* are less numerous than those who work on the material level. The gift is somewhat less common in the population, and the practitioner must go through a developmental period (*desarrollo*) that can be traumatic, or at least unsettling. Nevertheless, there is a growing movement of spiritualism in south Texas. This movement, and the practice of the *curandero* on this level, revolve around a belief in spirit beings who inhabit another plane of existence, but who are interested in making periodic contacts with the world. The *curandero* learns to become a link, a direct line of communication between this and that other world. In some cases the *curanderos* claim to have direct control over these spirit beings, and in other cases they merely act as a channel through which messages pass, much like a living telephone connection.

The heart of the spiritual movement in Mexican American communities lies in the activities of spiritual centers (*centros espiritistas*) that are staffed by trance mediums and others with occult abilities. This trend in visiting spiritualist centers appears to be relatively recent. It is not reported from the 1950s by Madsen (1964a), Rubel (1960, 1966), Clark (1959) and others who have done research on Mexican

American folk medicine. In addition, most of our older informants could remember when there were very few spiritualists practicing in the area.

Even though the practice of mediumship is relatively new among the Mexican Americans of south Texas, it is very ancient in other human societies. Mediumship is the ability to act as a communication link with the spiritual world. It is so widespread that a special term, 'shamanism,' has been attached to this practice to make it easier to compare the activities of shamans in one society to those in another and to avoid the negative connotations that have built up around the other labels associated with 'shaman,' such as 'witch doctor,' 'medicine man,' and 'spiritualist.' Michael Harner, working with shaman in Latin America, gives the following description of the group:

> A shaman may be defined as a man or woman who is in
> direct contact with the spirit world through a trance
> state and has one or more spirits at his command to
> carry out his bidding for good or evil. Typically, shamans
> bewitch persons with the aid of spirits or cure persons
> made ill by other spirits. . . . Depending on his traditions
> and beliefs, a shaman may also influence the course of
> events, find lost or stolen objects, define the identity of
> people who have committed crimes, communicate with
> the spirits of dead relatives and friends of clients, foretell
> the future, and practice clairvoyance. Contemporary an-
> thropology tends to view the shaman as a psychothera-
> pist, but the people of the cultures in which he operates
> believe him to be able to contact and deal with an invisi-
> ble spirit world. [Harner 1973 : xi–xii]

This definition fits both the shamans (*los mediums*) in Mexican American communities and the people's beliefs about them. The symbols and language they use can be viewed as the Mexican American cultural expression of a worldwide human phenomenon. This condition is clearly recognized by the *curanderos* themselves, especially those who belong to national and international organizations of spiritualists with memberships from various cultures around the world. These international groups periodically gather in a host country, like any other professional group, and exchange ideas and techniques. One of our informants went to one such meeting in Mexico while our research was in progress and was elated over the exchange of information there.

The practice of spiritualism rests on a belief called the soul concept. The soul concept is a belief in the existence of spirit beings, entities derived from once-living humans. The soul, then, is the immortal and immaterial component, the life and personality force of human beings. It continues in existence after physical death, but on a plane of reality separated from the physical world. This concept is important not only to *curanderismo* but also to the religious and mystical beliefs found in all Western cultures.

The soul is variously described by *curanderos* as a force field, an ectoplasm, concentrated vibrations, or a group of electrical charges that can exist separate from the physical body of human beings. It is thought to retain the personality, knowledge, and motivations of the individual, even after the death of the corporal body. Under the proper conditions the soul is believed to have the ability to contact and affect persons living in the physical world. While souls can occasionally be seen as ghosts or apparitions by ordinary human beings, they are more commonly thought to exist in the special spiritual realm. For some people this realm has various divisions that have positive or negative connotations (heaven, limbo, purgatory, and hell). Other people see the spiritual realm as a parallel to the physical world. They claim that the spiritual is a more pleasant plane to live on, but few attempt any suicidal test of this belief. One informant observed while discussing the spiritual level of *curanderismo*: "Those of us who have developed our abilities through the World Spiritual Doctrine call these [entities] spirits [*espiritos*], but actually spirits and souls [*animas*] are the same thing. In the past they were called souls, as our grandparents taught us, and now we call them spirits."

These spirits' activities closely parallel their former activities in this world. Since the personality, knowledge, and motivation of the spirits are much the same as they were for the living being, there are both good and evil spirits, spirits who heal and spirits who harm, wise spirits and fools.

Many of these spirits are thought to want to communicate with or act upon the physical plane. Some have left tasks undone in their physical lives and wish to complete them; others want to help or harm; many wish to communicate messages to friends and relatives, telling them of their happiness or discontent with their new existence. *Curanderos* with the ability to work on the spiritual realm therefore become the communication link between these two worlds. The impression that some *curanderos* give is that there are multitudes of spirits who want to communicate with the physical world. Those spirits tend to hover around those who have the gift to become a medium, waiting for an opportunity to enter their bodies and possess them. *Curanderos* use this circumstance to explain some of the cases of spirit possession in Western cultures by pointing out that those who become possessed are people with a strong potential to be trance mediums, but who have not had the opportunity to learn how to control this condition.

Only certain people have the gift (*el don*) to work on the spiritual level; however, this distinction is one of degree rather than kind. All people are felt to have the innate ability to receive spiritual communications, but it is more pronounced in some than in others, just as all human beings have the potential to speak, yet only a few become great orators.

The ability to become a medium is centered in the *cerebro*, that portion of the brain found at the base of the skull.

Those with the gift are said to have a more fully developed *cerebro*, while those without it are said to have a weak *cerebro* (*un cerebro debil*). This weakness has no relationship to either intelligence or character, only to the ability to communicate with the spiritual realm. Weak *cerebros* represent a danger for anyone who wishes to become a medium. One informant was warned about this problem.

> INFORMANT: My mother talked to her [a *curandera* working on the spiritual level] and all she said was that I didn't have the potential, or that if I did learn a few things, how to cure this and that, and I tried to perform it on someone that was ill, it [the illness] might rebound on me.
>
> QUESTIONER: She told you you could not do this? That it would rebound on you?
>
> INFORMANT: Yeah, I never asked why. Whatever she says goes. She said that if I ever get to the point where I did learn something pertaining to *curanderismo* and I tried to practice it on somebody else or tried to cure somebody, that it would rebound on me. So the best thing to do would be just to keep out of it.

In most cases, encounters with *curanderos* like the one described above appear to be sincere attempts on the part of practitioners to prevent people from doing harm to themselves, rather than attempts by the healers to limit the number of people practicing *curanderismo*. The danger mentioned is very real from their point of view, and not to warn someone about it would be a serious ethical lapse.

Only rare individuals demonstrate potential spontaneously and can use their gift without further training. So *curanderos* frequently test their clients and friends for the gift of healing, and those with this gift are generally encouraged to develop their ability. Potential mediums are discovered through this testing process and then, if they are willing, go through an extensive training process to learn how to use the gift. This testing and training takes many forms and is partially dependent on the knowledge, abilities, and personality of the *curandero* doing the testing.

During the course of our research, most of the members of the research team were tested for latent abilities by one or more *curanderos*. The *curanderos* did not have any known contact with one another and, interestingly enough, there was considerable agreement among them on both the existence of abilities in particular individuals and what those abilities were. This consistency strongly suggests that further research should be pursued in this area to uncover the basis for it.

The least elaborate test performed on the research team could be called a laying on of hands. We were ushered into a *curandera*'s workroom and sat on the day bed and chairs she had provided so we could talk with her. To prepare us for the test, she asked what our birth dates were, explaining that people born in certain months (rather than certain astrological signs) were more likely to develop healing powers than people born in other months. February and August were two of the months indicated as birth months for potential mediums. (Not all *curanderos* adhere to this theory, and in fact, one called it completely false—one indication of the considerable idiosyncratic diversity within the entire system.) She then began a prayer to the spirits (*los espiritos*), asking them to communicate with the research team. She went to each person, made the sign of the cross with a special oil (*acete de siete potentias*) on their foreheads, and clasped each of their heads with one of her hands on the forehead (*la frente*), the other at the base of the skull (*el cerebro*). She later explained that she concentrated on sensing the person's spirit between her hands. She said that she sent mental vibrations through the person's brain and the sensations she perceived are "normal," "tight," and "loose." It is persons with tight vibrations who she felt have the ability to concentrate and the potential to work in the spiritual realm.

The test performed by another *curandero* is interesting in its points of contrast to the one above. Rather than attempting a direct sensation of potential through a ritualized laying on of hands, this test depended upon contact with the spiritual realm to produce its results. Five members of the research team were at the home of a *curandero* who was establishing a new spiritual center in one of the towns in the area. After talking for some time about general topics, he asked if he could perform a test on the team. He explained that before attending a spiritual session, it is beneficial to know whether any of the participants have the potential to become a medium. If any of the participants possessed that gift, he would prefer to take precautionary measures to protect them from harm during the session.

To test the group he had everyone sit comfortably in a semicircle at one end of the room. Participants were instructed to remove all metal objects from direct contact with their bodies, not to cross their arms or legs at any time during the test, and to sit with their eyes closed. They were to sit with their hands resting on their laps, palms up, and to concentrate on a Supreme Being, "God or whatever else you want to call him," excluding all other thoughts. He told them, "Forget about everything else and concentrate on just that (the Supreme Being); afterwards, whatever you felt, you will tell me. It might be that you felt very light, as if you were floating or that you felt as if you were sinking. If you don't feel anything, then tell me you felt nothing."

He brought a clear glass filled with water and placed it upon a table beside him. He had the group sit silently and close their eyes. He stood beside the water glass making a silent invocation to the spirit realm. The test lasted for fifteen minutes. (For some of us the impulse to peek was nearly overwhelming at times and may have spoiled our concentration.) When the test was over, he asked the group to describe any sensations that were felt. The session was recorded on tape and two of the responses are translated below:

PARTICIPANT A: I felt I was going up and down three times. It was like when you're upside down and then turn all of a sudden and the blood rushes to your head. Like lifting up and then all of a sudden zooming down. One time I felt as if I were leaning, but I didn't.

CURANDERO: And you?

PARTICIPANT B: I felt an alternation of darkness and pressure. In the darkness I could see images. Either blood vessels or perhaps faces. The pressure was like too much light. It was brilliant.

CURANDERO: Did you feel your head nodding up and down?

PARTICIPANT B: Yes. I also heard a baby cry outside the house.

CURANDERO: There was no baby outside. That was in your mind. You nodded your head in answer to a question. I asked the spirits to indicate which of you have the faculties to be a medium. As soon as I asked the question, you began nodding.

PARTICIPANT B: It felt as if my head would slowly become lighter and lighter and would raise up. As soon as it got there, it would become heavier and slowly sink down. It was strange, because it felt like it was doing that by itself. That went on for some time.

CURANDERO: You were the only one who answered the question. [To another person] If he prepares himself correctly, he can become a very powerful medium. That's why his head bowed, it was to indicate an answer to that question.

The *curandero* then asked the other three persons present to describe their sensations. One had felt nothing, one had seen swirls of colors, and the other had felt slight differences in pressure. From similar tests on other groups conducted by one of the authors, these are apparently all common responses to sitting with your eyes closed for fifteen minutes concentrating on a Supreme Being. Only one individual out of this group was indicated to have the potential to be a medium. However, the *curandero* later discovered that another person present at that test had the potential to be a clairvoyant (*vidente*).

The researcher who was identified as a potential medium was offered the opportunity to apprentice to the *curandero*. This caused us to ask whether people neglect developing a gift. We were told that not everyone who is discovered to have a gift develops it, because there are a number of dangers and inconveniences that make the life of a *curandero* unattractive to potential healers.

Some people fear the social problems associated with becoming a *curandero*, while others are bothered by the element of supernatural danger involved. Many people discover they have the gift and ignore or even repress this information for fear of being set apart. One *curandero* said it thus: "Many people don't want to [become mediums] because of fear, of embarrassment, and many other things. They don't want to get involved because of their profession or their home life."

Curanderos are viewed from many different social perspectives within their communities. Some people seek them out as their sole or major health resource, while others view them as quacks, fakes, or even the Devil's emissaries on earth. All of these people view the *curandero* as a person set apart from the rest of humanity, either by his gifts or his actions. The *curandero* is considered different from ordinary people, and this difference produces respect, distrust, and even fear. Sometimes it produces the accusation that the *curandero* is a *brujo*, a witch, doing antisocial magic, so not everyone feels drawn to this profession.

Other people ignore the problem of being set apart but are concerned about the legality of *curanderismo*. The medical-practices acts of many states are written in such a way that *curanderismo* is potentially illegal. Some types of spiritual healing could possibly be construed as practicing medicine without a license. However, the practicing mediums reject this suggestion; from their viewpoint it is not they but spirits who perform the cures. Nevertheless, this problem causes some people to choose not to become *curanderos*.

Most people who decide not to become mediums do so because of the supernatural rather than the social dangers involved, yet the *curanderos* emphasize that there are also some dangers associated with having the gift and not using it. The primary danger, from the *curandero*'s perspective, is that the potential medium has a brain sensitive to spiritual communication and possession, yet does not know how to protect himself from spiritual intrusions. These problems were pointed out by one *curandero* before one of the researchers began training as a medium: "Many people have problems and don't know why, until they find they have these faculties. When you have this potential, there will be someone [spirits] pulling you to develop this thing you have. You can have many problems if you have this potential and do not develop it." The problems encountered, if the gift is very strong, run from possession at worst to frequent bad dreams at best.

The *curanderos* emphasized that the most vulnerable time for the medium comes during his development (*desarrollo*) when he has opened up new channels in his mind and does not yet know how to close them or protect himself. This is the main reason why it is necessary for the developing medium to be trained by another fully developed spiritualist. The developed spiritualist can place a "mantle of protection" over an apprentice until he is able to protect himself from harm. This potential harm has two sources, one human and one supernatural.

The human danger comes from other spiritualists, especially those working with evil spirits, in the dark realm (*trabajan en obscuro*). These people can sense the development of new mediums and sometimes attack them, either through magic on the material level or through agents in the spiritual realm. The reasons some *brujos* make these attacks are not clear. In part it seems to be done because of the rivalry that exists between those working "in the good" (*en lo bueno*) and those working "in the bad" (*en lo malo*); it may be that the attacker does not want other people practicing in his field. In most cases, unless the attacker is very powerful, the apprentice's teacher is easily able to counter these attacks, which usually come at night in the form of bad dreams.

A more serious danger exists in the spirit realm. There are few people who can develop the ability to become a medium, and according to the *curanderos* there are many, many spirits who want to make contact with the physical world. Some of these spirits are good; some are evil. According to the *curanderos*, they tend to fight for a chance to enter the apprentice's body. Without his teacher's protection, these spirits could take over the developing medium's body and create problems. They can, at the very least, exhaust the apprentice. These spirits can also physically harm the apprentice by causing him to fall from the chair during trance or to thrash about the room and injure himself. To counteract these problems, the teacher gives the apprentice mental strength and controls the spirit's access to him.

The early dangers that are a part of becoming a medium are not permanent. One protection is that at some point in their training the apprentices receive spiritual protectors that aid in their development and protect them both in and from the spirit realm. Two varieties of spiritual protectors were encountered during the course of the research project. Some of the spiritualists claimed famous persons as protectors, while others said that their protectors were simply appropriate individuals within the spirit realm. The method for contacting these protectors also varied.

Those people who claim to be spiritually protected by famous people frequently mention Don Pedrito Jaramillo, Niño Fidencio, Francisco Villa (Pancho Villa, revolution-

ary general in the 1910 Mexican revolution), and Emiliano
Zapata (another of the northern leaders in the 1910 revolution). Others claim their patron saint or their favorite saint
as a protector. Among the most common are San Martin de
Porres, San Martin Caballero, the Virgin of San Juan, and St.
Michael the Archangel. One such spiritualist gave the following directions for contacting a spiritual protector:

> You buy a crystal bowl. You take it to church and you
> ask the priest to bless it for you. Then you fill the bowl
> with water in your home or wherever you have it, and
> you speak into it. You will say: "In the name of the Fa-
> ther, the Son and the Holy Spirit; God the Father; God
> the Son; God the Holy Spirit; dear brother (name of spirit
> you are contacting) give me your spiritual strength and
> protection." Then the spirit will direct you and in return
> you will give it respect. The spirit will tell you what
> recipe you are going to use and what you are going to
> cure. You can't really start to work until you have this
> protection.

The individuals who did not have famous protectors
stated that they encountered their protectors during the development of their faculties (*desarrollo*). A particular spirit
would return from one trance session to the next and would
eventually announce to the medium that he or she was to
be a protector. From that time on, that spirit protects the
medium.

A developing medium of this type normally receives at
least two protectors during his training. They become spiritual gatekeepers: during the medium's trance they are in
charge of protecting his body while his spirit is away from it.
They choose which spirits will enter the body and how long
they stay, and they call back the medium's spirit at the end
of the trance. Without this spiritual protection, it is said that
the medium could not work in the spirit realm. On other occasions, these protectors also teach and give the medium in-

struction on curing or supernatural knowledge that he could not find in books or from other mediums. This is especially important because once the medium has full control over his gift, the *curandero* who is his teacher normally withdraws the protection given to the developing medium, and the new *curandero* is on his own. He is expected to protect himself from attacks against him from either the physical or the spiritual realm. In most cases he is expected to defend himself through his knowledge, his mental strength, and the help of his protectors. However, spiritualists and other *curanderos* do sometimes form groups for mutual protection and to share knowledge.

The spirit realm usually cannot be reached through a normal state of consciousness. Contact comes through dreams or when a *curandero* goes into a trance. Both of these states are altered states of consciousness—states when the mind is receptive, according to the *curanderos*, to contact with the spirit world.

Contact with spirits through dreams is not uncommon within *curanderismo*. One *curandera* said, "Spirits work with or give waking manifestations to people who are not scared. With those who would be frightened, they usually communicate in dreams." She also stated that if you have this gift, "you may hear voices at night . . . or have a revelation. If so, you can put a glass of water, a rosary, and a crucifix at the head of your bed so that you will not be frightened by these manifestations. The spirits know who is scared by these things and who isn't; they work with each in the way that best suits that person's needs."

The most common way a *curandero* works with the spirit world is not through dreams, but in a trance. This trance state is something that he learns during his training to become a medium. It is a form of controlled possession. The *curanderos* stated that the medium allows spirits to take possession of his body—to control his hands, his legs, his mouth, and to use his body to communicate with people in the physical world.

From the perspective of the observer, the trance begins as the *curandero* sits, eyes closed, and begins to breathe heavily. Sometimes the body sags, then returns upright as a spirit "takes possession of the body." When these spirits "come down" upon the *curandero*, a number of changes often take place. The facial expression of the medium changes, as does his body posture, and each spirit supposedly attempts to conform the medium's body as closely as possible to its own former physical appearance and mannerisms. Thus, a man with a crippled arm in life would hold the arm of the *curandero*'s body in as close an approximation to his old physical appearance as possible. The same practice holds true for other physical mannerisms, such as a woman plucking at her dress, a man brushing his whiskers, or another petting a dog that had accompanied him into the spiritual realm.

The *curanderos* explained these changes by stating that as the medium goes into trance his own spirit leaves his body and another enters to take over the vacated shell. When asked where they go, most informants answered vaguely. However, they usually said that they project their spirits into another place and that they remain conscious throughout this travelling process and can remember everything that they see or hear while they are gone from their bodies. The only place most *curanderos* felt the soul is not allowed to go without special preparation and strength is within the room where the physical body rests. Therefore, they say they normally have no knowledge of what happened there, since their spirit was somewhere else during the trance.

Wherever the personality that belongs to the *curandero* in a waking state goes, the personalities or spirits that present themselves in the trance state are normally considerably different. Individual spirits can be distinguished by changes in speech patterns, voice quality, and physical mannerisms. A medium, regardless of sex, may speak with the voice of a man, woman, or child. Preliminary observations indicate that there are differences in the choice of words and word patterns between those of the spirit and those of the *curandero*. However, none of these changes are complete; there is always a recognizable element of the *curandero* in the spirit being. The healers attribute this to the fact that the spirits never gain absolute control over the body, and an element of the original owner always remains. The possessing spirit could never be attuned to the body as well as the body's own spirit, a circumstance that affords some natural protection to the personality of the healer, which might otherwise be displaced by the possessing spirit.

The trance ends when the possessing spirit leaves the medium's body, the medium again breathes heavily, and his own spirit returns without any knowledge of what went on in the room while he was gone.

Most *curanderos* must undergo training to learn to achieve and control the trance state. This training can proceed in a number of ways, and upon very rare occasions a person can spontaneously become an adept medium without outside help. These people may go through a series of trance states and learn without help to control these states and to cure. More frequently the developing medium, upon discovery of his gift, either goes to a spiritual center (*centro espiritista*) and receives development or is trained by a *curandero* who can work on the spiritual level. While the training is reported to be similar in both cases, the only developmental sessions directly observed during our research were the *curandero*-apprentice type; it is that process that is reported here.

This training, called *desarrollo*, is a gradual process of increasing the apprentice's contact with the spirit world, giving him more and more experiences in controlled trances and possessions, together with the knowledge necessary to develop and protect himself. The teacher is also responsible for not giving the apprentice knowledge so fast that he harms himself. For example, one apprentice, a member of the research team, came across a voodoo doll that had been shown to a colleague, so he asked the *curandero* what he should do if he found such objects.

CURANDERO: When you come up with something like that the best thing to do would be to tear it apart. There is a formula that you use as you tear the thing apart that will stop the harm from being done. Then, you should burn it after you tear it apart. You do several conjurings [*conjuros*] on it and it starts disintegrating until everything is burned.

APPRENTICE: Can you be harmed by handling it?

CURANDERO: No, not if the harm is directed at another person.

APPRENTICE: Can you tell me the words?

CURANDERO: Later I can, but not right now. I could tell you the words that you use and you could say them, but the person who is doing the evil would find out and would attack you if you didn't know how to protect yourself.

APPRENTICE: Okay, so how do I learn to protect myself?

CURANDERO: You need to develop yourself completely, so you can deal in other things [other forms of psychic energy and magic]. That way you will learn to protect yourself in every case, what to do in each instance. After you develop yourself, the spirits will give you a formula on how to protect yourself. Then, later on you will be able to use this knowledge along with different materials to defend yourself. Many people think these things are unimportant, but they are important. You have to be prepared.

Thus, the apprentice is encouraged to learn, but in the proper order and under the control of the *curandero*. After one step of the process has been mastered, he can move on to the next, learn new skills, and develop his powers in a logical manner.

Developing to be a medium is a highly personal, very idiosyncratic process. The *desarrollo* does not follow exactly the same course for any two developing mediums because their experiences are subjective impressions of an altered state of consciousness. These impressions are affected by the cultural expectations and experiences of the individual's mind. In addition, they must be described in a language that does not have the precise vocabulary to adequately handle these types of impressions; therefore, some of the things the apprentice experiences are simply indescribable.

Before the research began, several *curanderos* warned us that some things within the spiritual level could not be seen, heard, touched, or smelled in any ordinary sense. They could only be experienced. The following section should be read with these limitations in mind. It presents three perspectives on the process of development an apprentice goes through to become a medium. The information was gathered through direct participant observation and is given from the perspective of the observer, the *curandero,* and the internal perspective of the apprentice himself.

The *desarrollo* sessions are held one, two, or more times a week, depending on the availability of the *curandero* and the apprentice. Each session lasts from one to two hours, only a portion of which is devoted to the trance state. As in all other events within the Mexican American system of folk medicine, a high premium is placed on the social aspects of human relationships during the *desarrollo* sessions. The apprentice goes to the *curandero's* house or workroom, and they sit and visit. There is no rigid formality at these sessions and to begin immediately, without social discourse, would be considered rude and abrupt. Therefore, the topics of conversation in these initial visits (*pláticas*) range from current events, politics, art, and hobbies, to events in the lives of friends and family. The actual development begins only after the principals have sat, relaxed, and talked as friends. There is no element of superiority and inferiority in these sessions. The teacher regards the apprentice as a social equal. There are differences of knowledge, power, and assurance between them, but not inequalities in social status. The apprentice is approached as one who is invited, not forced, to learn.

When the visiting has reached a certain point, the *curandero* indicates it is time to begin the actual *desarrollo*. To protect the apprentice from hitting his head should he fall during the trance, the *curandero* moves a wooden chair into the center of the room, away from all other furniture. A wooden chair is used because the *curandero* guides the *desarrollo* by using two psychic forces, spiritual currents (*corrientes spirituales*) and mental vibrations (*vibraciones mentales*). The *curanderos* said that a metal chair or any metal object in contact with the individual in trance could cause mild electrical shocks when the *curandero* concentrates these forces on the apprentice. Therefore, mediums always sit on wooden chairs, which are nonconducting, and remove watches, rings, glasses and any other metal objects in contact with their body. The glasses are removed even if they are not metal because it is believed that the psychic energy can shatter them or they can be broken if the apprentice falls.

On the *curandero*'s desk or altar is a crystal bowl of prepared water (*agua preparada*) that has had special incantations said over it to give it special magnetic properties (*propiedades magneticas*). To prepare himself for the trance, the apprentice dips his hands in the water and rubs it on his forehead (*la frente*) and his *cerebro*. This necessary step was explained in the following way during an early research session:

RESEARCHER: Why do you have him put the water on his forehead and the *cerebro*?

CURANDERO: That is to protect him and to help him develop.

RESEARCHER: Do you put it on in a certain manner or do you simply put it on?

CURANDERO: You simply put it on.

RESEARCHER: You don't put it in the form of a cross or something like that?

CURANDERO: No, you just put it on. Anyone who is developing or developed puts it on for protection.

After putting on the *agua preparada,* the apprentice sits on the chair in a comfortable position. His feet rest on the floor, and his forearms rest on his lap. His hands rest on top of his knees, with palms upward and fingers gently curling. In this position, the apprentice is able to relax and begin to go into trance.

As the apprentice is going into trance the *curandero* stands in front of him, feet slightly spread and arms held out at his sides at nearly a forty-five-degree angle, and in the same plane as his body. He holds his palms facing toward the apprentice and speaks invocations (either silently or aloud) to the spirit realm. These invocations are said to protect the apprentice during trance and to call down or invite benevolent spirits to possess him.

To the observer, the apprentice goes in trance by closing his eyes and relaxing. His breathing becomes regular and deep. He tends to sag forward, bowing his head and bending at the waist, perhaps even bobbing or swaying slightly. He suddenly sits bolt upright, assuming a posture and facial expression noticeably different from the ones he normally has. When the apprentice sits up, the *curandero* says, it is because the first spirit has descended upon him and the development session has fully begun. *Curanderos* also indicate that other spirits are clustered around him waiting for a turn at possession.

The *curandero* takes water from his bowl (*copa*) with his left hand and sprinkles a circle of prepared water completely around the apprentice. This forms a protective circle, a barrier which prevents other spirits from reaching the developing medium. This limits the number of spirits that can descend on him and provides him with some protection against malevolent spirits during a particularly vulnerable time. The spirits can reportedly cross the barrier to leave the area but cannot reenter once they are beyond it.

From the apprentice's perspective, he begins the trance by sitting and relaxing. (The *curandero* has previously told him to concentrate in much the same way he did for the testing procedures). He closes his eyes and begins to breathe deeply. Colors, muted purples mixed with greens and occasional sky blues, often swirl in front of his eyes. Focusing on these colors helps his concentration and within a few seconds a slight feeling of remoteness descends upon him. This feeling creates conflicting sensations. On the one hand, he feels as if he can stand slightly back from himself and observe his own actions as an outsider. On the other hand, he begins to feel sensations in his body that suggest he should shift his posture, should make certain gestures, should move. The spirit that is presenting itself controls the body much as a puppet is controlled. This gives the apprentice the dual sensation of being able to observe and feel what is happening. These sensations go beyond simple kinetic perceptions. Two sensations generally present themselves first, a combination of sex and age. Weight is the next, combined with particular physical features. Yet writing them as a sequence is misleading, since they present themselves more rapidly than the sequence could be read. These sensations are heightened by concentration. To concentrate, the apprentice closes his mind to intruding, extraneous thoughts. With proper concentration, the apprentice has the sensation of being inhabited by someone else, while a small part of his mind remains as an observer of this process. According to the *curanderos*, if the apprentice wishes to achieve a complete trance state, he must learn to send this watchdog portion of his mind out of his body. Only then will the trance and possession be complete.

These sensations can persist for a long or a short time.

During these contacts the developing medium feels himself move, smile, write, gesture, or go through a number of other actions. Then, it is as if someone cut the strings on the puppet, and he sags and breathes deeply once again. The feeling of remoteness remains, but the sensation of another personality goes away almost as if it were pulled out of him by an unknown hand. After this, the process begins again with new sensations, gestures, and activities.

Early in his *desarrollo*, the apprentice cannot talk while in trance, but he frequently gestures, or even writes (with either hand). The writing, although different from his own, remains similar from session to session, according to which spirit is making the writing. Some spirits tend to repeat visits from session to session, especially those who have decided to aid the development of the apprentice or to become his protectors. Each new spirit that "comes down" on the apprentice during the trance session can be recognized by its particular posture, facial expressions, gestures, writing, and, later, voice and speech patterns.

From the perspective of the observer, all of this activity looks even more like a puppet adopting different characters, each with his own postures, gestures, sex, weight, and age. One character may be proud, another prim, another crippled, another fat. A steady progression of mute personalities is presented to the observer's view. Occasionally an earlier character presents itself for a second time. From session to session there are both repeating characters and new ones. Some present themselves for a very short time. Others remain and try to communicate. It is not unusual for a spirit to try to speak, but these early attempts are normally unsuccessful. This speech is generally inaudible or mumbly because the apprentice becomes interested in what is going to be said, loses concentration, and in the process makes it impossible for the spirit to speak. Often the apprentice feels as if his jaw were being massaged during these attempts. According to the *curandero*, these sensations are a sign that the spirits are preparing the body for the ability to speak.

APPRENTICE: My jaws hurt.

OBSERVER: He is preoccupied with not being able to talk.

CURANDERO: The time will come when he will begin to speak. There are mediums who on the fourth or fifth development begin to speak, and there are others who will not speak until the twentieth or twenty-fifth development. Those are good indications which he is getting. The sore jaw means that he is being given massages so that he will be able to speak soon.

It is not uncommon for the spirits to write messages long before they can speak. To the apprentice, this writing feels as if his hand is moving of its own accord. In fact, if he concentrates on the writing it often becomes illegible, or he intrudes his own words or nonsense syllables on the messages. If he relaxes the hand as much as possible, identifiable words and messages come out. One interesting feature about this writing is that each spirit writes consistently with either its right or left hand. Therefore, in the course of one *desarrollo* session, the apprentice may write messages with both hands, regardless of which hand he normally uses for writing. As the development of the new medium progresses, his ability to write and speak improves. The *curanderos* explain that the spirits must open new channels in the body and brain, so it is to be expected that practice and exposure would enhance the spirits' ability to use the body and the body's ability to respond.

To the *curandero*, this process is one in which he encourages and aids the apprentice's spirit to disassociate itself from his material body. Spirits present themselves to him, clustering around the apprentice. Some simply stand by, some descend on and begin developing the apprentice. The *curandero* perceives all of these spirits and can describe their appearance. He can even feel whether they are related to the neophyte. One *curandero* described a spirit that he perceived during a *desarrollo* session. Note the ambiguous nature of the description, although the *curandero* and the apprentice agreed on the sex of the spirit without prior communication:

> CURANDERO: I think it was a spirit who is related to him.
> OBSERVER: Was it a woman?
> CURANDERO: He doesn't know him. He was just at his side.
> OBSERVER: What did he look like?
> CURANDERO: He's tall. He's a little bit taller than [the apprentice].
> APPRENTICE: It couldn't be my father then. He's shorter than I am.
> CURANDERO: To me it is a relative of his. That other one that presented himself [at an earlier session] was also a relative of his. But this one isn't old. This one is younger.

If the developed medium tires during the *desarrollo*, the *curandero* often lights a candle to give him further mental strength. After a series of spirits have presented themselves, the apprentice comes out of trance. The apprentice's ability to remain disassociated from his body rapidly diminishes, the dual sensations go away, and as he opens his eyes he feels normal once again. To the observer, the last spirit or personality leaves, the apprentice sags one last time, then sits up with his normal posture, opens his eyes, and gets up from the chair. The *curandero* says that he brings about this ending. He recalls the neophyte's spirit, causes the other spirits to leave, and brings the neophyte out of trance and back to a normal state of reality.

The session does not end here, however. The *curandero* takes the time to probe the sensations of the apprentice during the trance, to assess how his *desarrollo* is progressing, and to answer the apprentice's questions and doubts. This session begins with the apprentice relating what each spirit and sensation felt like when it descended on him.

APPRENTICE: At the beginning, just before the first one presented herself, I felt a very bright light. It was pure white, like flash. Then, I felt a lot of heat on one side of my face, and a smell; something between candles and skin.

CURANDERO: Well, the heat could be the respiration of the spirits. That is natural. The smell thing is natural too. When you are developed you have all of those faculties.

APPRENTICE: The first one to come down was a woman. She is crippled on her left side. I could feel myself leaning that way, as if there was no support in my side. I just bent over and couldn't stop. I stopped when my head almost touched the floor on that side. Then I sat back up.

OBSERVER: He brought you back up.

APPRENTICE: How?

OBSERVER: I don't know. All he did was to stretch out his hand, hold it about two feet from your head. Then he moved it in an arch. As he moved his hand upward, you sat back up. He didn't touch you, but you sat up at the same speed he moved his hand.

APPRENTICE: It felt as if a pressure had been removed and I had support in that side again. Did he do something to the room?

OBSERVER: No.

APPRENTICE: The room became very bright when we first started out. In fact, it was so bright that it was hard to concentrate.

The *curandero* does not always explain what each sensation means, saying that each medium, as he develops, becomes more sensitive to his environment and that the apprentice must expect to encounter odd sensations such as bright light, noises, changes in pressure in a room and other sensations associated with his developing powers. For example, the *curandero* explained one action the apprentice found disturbing:

> APPRENTICE: The first day I was here I sat on that chair and felt very uncomfortable, so I went and sat on another chair. Why was that?
>
> CURANDERO: Many people who come to see me have serious problems. When a person sits on a chair, he leaves an impression on it. So, when you sat there you picked up those impressions. It happens because of the faculty you have. As soon as you sat on the chair you got all of the sensations that people have left when they sit in that chair. Since you are becoming sensitive to people's problems, you felt uncomfortable and you moved.

At the end of these *desarrollo* sessions, the talk reverts to social conversation for a time before the apprentice takes his leave. This developmental process continues, with variations, until the apprentice is a fully developed medium.

Fully developed mediums have some control over how, where, and when they work. Some mediums work alone. Some may work only on family problems, while others may work only for their own knowledge and gratification. Others work in groups with other mediums and with other persons who supposedly have spiritual or psychic powers. And some mediums work in elaborate spiritual centers (*centros espiritistas*) that are formal spiritual churches, often dedicated to a particular spirit (Niño Fidencio or Francisco Rojas, for example). The spiritual centers and the activities surrounding them take on all of the major attributes of a formalized religion.

Many *curanderos* with abilities to work on the spiritual level of healing prefer to work at home alone. Their practices tend to be less uniform than the practices of mediums working at spiritual centers, since they do not have to conform to a calendar or the ritual structure of the formalized temples. However, there is enough uniformity in their actions to allow an accurate description. One healer is described from the perspective of a college student in his early twenties who was one of her clients. This particular *curandera* had been handling problems for him and his family for several years.

RESEARCHER: Can you describe how this *curandera* works, in as great detail as you can?

STUDENT: We drive up into the driveway of a fairly decent-looking place. She walks out and greets us, shakes our hands, asks how we are doing and how we have been. Then we go inside. She's got a small room from about here to the wall, perhaps eight by ten feet. She has an altar with saints and candles and flowers on it. She has a small vase, shaped like a crystal ball, sitting on a table. Sometimes it has water in it and sometimes it's turned upside down.

You walk in there and sit down and she's talking with you. She's not in her trance, it's just social talk. Then she sits and puts her hand on that crystal deal. She taps it, closes her eyes, and she starts asking you what kind of problem you have or whatever you want to ask her.

RESEARCHER: Her voice changes?

STUDENT: Yes it does. It's a lot lower. All of a sudden her voice becomes soft, sort of like whispering. Really mild.

RESEARCHER: Does she keep her hands on the glass all of the time?

STUDENT: No. Sometimes she grabs a folder with papers in it and starts writing down things on it, using her finger.

RESEARCHER: Can she read what she has written?

STUDENT: I'm pretty sure she can.

RESEARCHER: How does she cure people?

STUDENT: She does it in a number of ways. Some time ago my mother had pains on both of her heels. She went to the doctor and the doctor didn't find anything wrong. So she went over to this lady again, who said it was something [a *trabajo* or hex] that [a woman across the alley from his house] had put in the yard. When my mother's out hanging up clothes, she's barefooted and she stepped on it. And that's what was hurting her. So [the *curandera*] gave her a shot on her arm like a regular shot. And that cured her.

RESEARCHER: How did she give her the shot?

[*The student simulates the action of giving an injection without a syringe or hypodermic.*]

RESEARCHER: Could your mother feel it?

STUDENT: She told me she didn't. But it cured her.

The informant went on to tell of several other cures this *curandera* had performed for his family. She had prescribed herbs, suggested the use of perfumes to ward off *enbidia* (envy) against the family from their neighbors, and suggested that the mother perform a series of *barridas* on her son-in-law to remove a hex against him that was making him ill and keeping him from work. Each of these cures could just as easily have been suggested or performed by a *curandero* working on the material level of *curanderismo*, but she did it from a trance. Therefore, what sets this *curandera* apart from those working strictly on the material level is not the tools she uses or the rituals she suggests to her clients, but the *source* of her diagnosis and cures, her contact with the spirit world.

Another very different type of mediumship occurs where the trance session is open to more than one person at the same time. This is a form of group session that can be carried out by a lone *curandero*, but is more often found at spiritual centers. While we were conducting research for this book we participated in a newly developing spiritual center in a small border town in south Texas. During the research period, the center started out as a place for a well-known Mexican *curandero* (from Reynosa) to come across the border one day a week and provide services to the people in that town. Gradually, a group of people came together and the *curandero* began to work there on the spiritual level, and a nucleus for a new center began to form around the *curandero*.

The medium held the spiritual sessions in a flower and gift shop wedged tightly between a pool hall on one side and a beer joint on the other. The songs of the juke box and the clicking of the pool balls could always be heard in the background as the spiritual session progressed. The session was held in the back room of the shop, since it was the only room that could accommodate from twelve to twenty or more persons sitting, somewhat widely spaced, in a circle.

These spiritual sessions were held on Tuesday nights, and the events at these sessions always followed an orderly pattern. About an hour before the session was scheduled to begin, the regular members of the spiritual group began to gather at the store, standing or sitting in small groups in the front room or the workroom (but seldom in the back room where the session would be held). The members generally brought with them family members and friends who were having problems and wished to be cured. Others came out of curiosity.

These sessions always began with a period of social visiting and conversation. During this preliminary period the *curandero* managed to talk with nearly every individual and family present. These were social conversations rather than consultations, and always seemed to reassure people and make them more comfortable.

When the *curandero* finally decided it was time to begin, he would indicate that people should begin to gather in the back room. The woman who owned the store would shepherd the guests in while all of the regular members of the spiritual group were dressing. Members were encouraged to wear white, symbolizing working with spirits of the light, so they would put on robes they had made for these sessions. Meanwhile the others moved chairs, benches, and a day bed into a circle.

The *curandero* always sat in one corner of the room with the circle of chairs bulging out in front of him. To his right was a chair for his apprentice, to his left an altar with a jar of *agua preparada*, brought from his office. Cut flowers, preferably red ones, were often placed on the altar at the request of one of the spirits that came down during one of the early sessions.

When all had gathered and seated themselves on their chairs, the *curandero* began the session by giving detailed instructions to the group, because there were frequently new people and visitors present who would not know the proper behavior. The people were asked to remove all metal objects from contact with their bodies, because the cures during these sessions use what the *curandero* called spiritual currents (*corrientes espirituales*) and mental vibrations (*vibraciones mentales*). The *curandero* explained that when these currents and vibrations flow through metal that is in contact with the skin they can produce mild electrical shocks, which can disturb the patient and interrupt the cure. People were also asked to remove their glasses because a buildup of these forces is thought to be capable of shattering glass. The people were instructed not to cross their arms and legs during the trance. This has the effect of increasing the intensity of the vibrations in the area, making it uncomfortable for the spirit present in the body of the medium.

Occasionally, people attend the sessions who unknowingly possess some mediumistic potential, and they may fall into trance spontaneously during the session. For this reason the *curandero* always gives the group instructions on what to do if any of them should feel themselves falling into trance. They are instructed to cross their thumbs diagonally across the palms of their hands with their fingers extended straight out. Then they are to cross their arms, with their hands held in this position, across their chest. This action breaks the incipient trance. If the person fails to do this and falls into trance, he can be brought back by calling his name three times or by splashing water on him in the form of a cross.

After the instructions were given, the *curandero* prepared himself for the trance by rubbing *agua preparada* on his forehead and *cerebro* and having his apprentice do the same. The participants prepared themselves by dipping their hands in water with rose petals and rubbing it on their foreheads. The lights were turned out, a candle lit, and an invocation to the spirits read. This invocation said that the purpose of the session was to contact good spirits (*espiritos de la luz*). It asked that the good spirits protect the medium and the people present from evil spirits and evil influences throughout the trance.

While this invocation was being read, the *curandero* went into his trance. By the time the invocation, which takes about five minutes to read, was complete, he was in trance and the first spirit made its presence known to the group. Several spirits generally come down on the medium during these sessions and each is marked by changes in the medium's voice, posture, gestures, and facial expressions. The following brief transcription from one of these sessions reflects the feeling and activity present at a spiritual session in a developing temple where there is a considerable dialogue between the spirits and the participants.

1ST SPIRIT: *Buenas noches* [*in the voice of a male*].

This spirit was merely preparing the way for a second one to arrive and did no more than announce his presence and give the name of the spirit to come next. He soon left, and

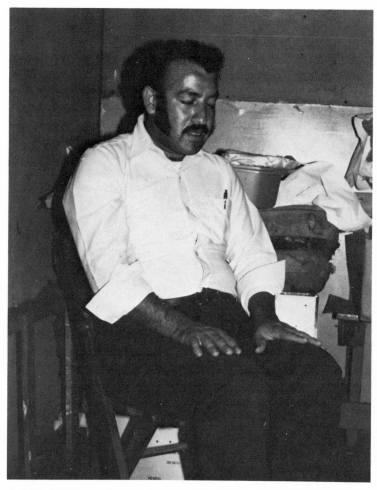

Spiritualist in trance during a spiritual session (*Photograph by Antonio Rivera*)

afterwards the second announced his presence. This second spirit was present to instruct the members on the way to prepare the spiritual center.

2ND SPIRIT: Good evening.

PARTICIPANTS: Good evening and welcome. Who are you, *hermano*?

2ND SPIRIT: A poor one, like you.

PARTICIPANTS: Welcome, we are pleased to make your acquaintance.

2ND SPIRIT: You will wear white at these sessions. . . . Bring flowers and water. . . . The flowers must be natural flowers. . . . They should be red or pink.

The second spirit instructed the people to place water in a large container so it could be blessed by the spirit coming next, Padre Elias. The second spirit said that Padre Elias was responsible for baptizing those present into the spiritual realm with this water and would be giving the regular members of the group their spiritual names and their duties and positions in the temple.

2ND SPIRIT: Padre Elias will give you a spiritual baptism. . . . Those who want and accept this baptism will be given spiritual marks and spiritual names. . . . You will receive a protector [*hermano guardian*]. . . . This is a voluntary thing.

PARTICIPANTS: Everything in the name of the Father we accept, *hermano*.

This spirit left and was replaced by a female spirit, who explained that the people had done some things wrong when the *curandero* had seemed to be in trouble in an earlier session.

3RD SPIRIT: Never touch him [the medium].

PARTICIPANTS: Okay.

3RD SPIRIT: Never touch him.

PARTICIPANTS: No, no, we won't touch him.

3RD SPIRIT: Put water on him, talk to him, but don't touch him. He is protected any way and nothing will happen to him. I am leaving. I only came by to say hello and because you called me.

PARTICIPANTS: We are very grateful that you look over [the medium] and us.

3RD SPIRIT: When I am called, I come. Goodbye.

PARTICIPANTS: Goodbye.

The next spirit that came down was Padre Elias. His voice was stronger than the other spirits; it seemed to fill up the room. His speeches were much longer and more forcefully given than the others, much like sermons in church with many allusions and symbols.

PADRE ELIAS: I want to explain some things before I baptize you. The road for helping our Father is very steep and very narrow. At your sides, many doors will open offering you anything you want. But you have to know which door to open. Seven doors will be placed in front of you, but you will find truth behind only one. Behind the others, you will find suffering, shame, and tears. The long and narrow road is the only true way. You can find riches and many beautiful things, but you will have to pay for them in the end.

PARTICIPANTS: But God will put goodness in our hearts, so we will know how to choose so that we will know the truth and understand it?

PADRE ELIAS: The door to our Father is very small and very narrow and very few will be able to fit through it. No matter how narrow it is, you will be able to fit through it if you make the right choice. Depending on the road you have chosen, you will know how to choose between the door of pleasure, between the door of vice, the door of knowledge, all in front of the door of truth.

Your choice depends on you alone. In this ideal time of grace you will be given things according to the will of the Father. And that which you give him will be received. Look well at what you are going to give him. Money is not acceptable. You do not give him gifts, but truth. That is all. And as it is given, so it will be received. At the same time, your acts will be considered and according to this you will keep on receiving. Remember one thing, no one reaches the Father without purifying the spirit. The material things you will leave here. The spiritual things are the only ones that reach our Father. You can wash a dress and get the stains out. The soul and spirit cannot be washed. They will be presented to the Father as they are. It is up to you whether they get there stained or clean.

Meditate on what I have told you. I am going to retire for a few minutes so you can do so.

At this point the spirit left for a few minutes, then returned.

PADRE ELIAS: I have come back, *hermanos*. Have you meditated?

PARTICIPANTS: Yes.

PADRE ELIAS: I have presented these roads so you might understand them. Are you disposed to receive this spiritual mark? If you have any questions, ask them.

PARTICIPANTS: What is there that awaits us after all of this?

PADRE ELIAS: A question will be answered with another question. In what way can our Father serve you?

PARTICIPANTS: In all ways.

PADRE ELIAS: Your answer was the answer I wanted.

He then proceeded to the baptism. Beginning on the right side of the medium, as he faced inward into the circle, he had each person who was willing come forward, and with the water made available earlier, he baptized each into the spiritual realm, giving each a spiritual name and protector. One example follows:

PADRE ELIAS: Give me your hands. Blessed are you who are lending your services and brain so that God's will will be accomplished. With Joshua's (*Josue*) name you

will be received into our spiritual world. You invoke
his spirit to protect you from whatever worries you
have or whatever difficulty you meet. He will answer
your plea as your guide and protector. Because in his
name you have been baptized in a state of grace.

Each participant was then asked to dip fingers into *agua
preparada* and to make a cross on his forehead and on his
cerebro. After each volunteer passed by the medium being
baptized, blessed, and given a new name, each was given a
new duty in the temple.

This activity is apparently common in newly forming
spiritual temples, and instructions to the participants continue to be a part of the temple functions, in a modified
form called *cátedras* or sermons, in even the most formalized
spiritual centers. This particular ceremony marked the beginning of the transition from a loosely associated group to
an incipient temple. At this point the *curandero* began more
actively seeking potential mediums (along with clairvoyants
and others with psychic ability) who would normally form
the nucleus of the temple. In the case of this group, however, no charismatic leader developed, nor were enough people found willing to develop their abilities to keep the
temple well staffed. Since the *curandero* could not and
would not be the only medium in the temple and since the
people could not find a place for a temple that was not used
for mundane purposes that would interfere with its uses as a
temple, this incipient temple eventually folded and the people returned to seeking the *curandero*'s advice on an individual basis.

Five to eight different spirits normally presented themselves through the medium at the spiritual sessions in the
incipient temple. Some were instructors like Padre Elias,
and some were announcers, preparing the way for others,
much as if they were announcing nobility at a court function. Some appeared merely to be interested in visiting with

the participants to banter and match wits with them, providing comic relief in an otherwise serious atmosphere. In a number of sessions a witty, comic spirit appeared just after the brief appearance of an evil spirit. This threatening spirit always frightened the members of the group into almost rigid inactivity, then jeered at them because they were unable to defend themselves from his presence. The witty spirit provided much-needed relief from the evil spirit's taunts.

From the point of view of the participants, the most important spirits who presented themselves at these sessions were the healing spirits. They were the ones whom the participants came to interact with, and, for most people, the other spirits were of relatively little importance. The healing spirits always asked those who had problems to come forward to speak with them. This is one of the few times during these sessions that people were allowed to move about inside the circle. Each person with a problem came forward and stood just in front of the seated medium. The medium then grasped the patient's hand or wrist with his forefinger and thumb encircling the wrist. With his eyes remaining closed at all times, the medium sometimes stood with one hand on the patient's forehead and another at the *cerebro*, searching the patient's mind with currents and vibrations that would pinpoint the problem. When this examination was finished, the spirit suggested cures. The cures often combined herbal remedies, magical formulas, rituals, and promises of direct spiritual intervention to solve the problem. Sometimes the patients were asked to return for further instructions, while others were told their problems would go away immediately.

At the end of each spiritual session, which often lasted two to three hours, the final spirit would indicate the termination of the session and the imminent return of the medium's spirit. A closing prayer was read by participants at that point, thanking the spirits for their aid and attention.

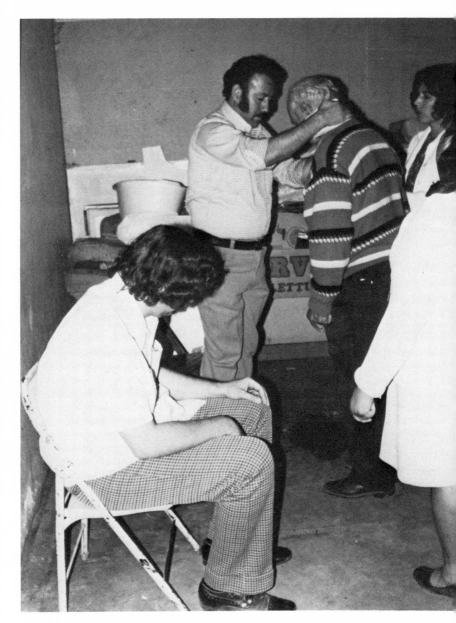

Spiritualist healing a participant in a spiritual session *(Photograph by Antonio Rivera)*

After the medium came out of trance during the reading of the prayer, the lights were turned back on and people once again began social conversations, interspersed with discussion of all of the events that occurred during the spiritual session. Someone would always take time to relate the events of the evening to the medium, who said he had no memory of what occurred in the room while his spirit was out of his body. Within a half hour or so the participants would take leave of the *curandero* and other members of the group and depart for home.

Solitary mediums like the ones described above are in a vulnerable position. They feel that they are open to attack from both the physical world and the spiritual realm. If other *curanderos* are jealous or dislike them, they may be magically attacked and have only their own strength and knowledge to protect them; or evil spirits may decide to gain control of their minds, and the mediums and their protectors must have the strength to overcome such attacks. This is one of the reasons that mediums tend to band together in loose associations or even formal, international organizations.

The loose associations are based on friendship and geographical proximity. One *curandera* explained, "I have friends that protect me. They check on me [periodically] and if they see something is going to happen to me, they light a candle and pray for me. Or I receive a spiritual message and I pray for them. Then nothing goes wrong for them." This kind of association often grows up between the teacher and the apprentice and even extends to other apprentices the teacher has had.

The larger associations of mediums working within the spiritual centers are much more formalized. In some cases, these groups perform functions similar to those of a licensing body. One informant described these associations as they exist in Mexico, near the border:

It is similar to a doctor who cannot work without licensing. All the mediums in the temples belong to a group. They have proof that they belong to an association of spirituals.

One woman, for example, founded a center because she started working at another center and discovered she could cure. So she became a member of a spiritual association in Mexico and asked for permission to start her own center. To prove that she belongs to the group, she has a picture of all of the people who belong to the association. It is large. Eight hundred to nine hundred people belong.

These associations protect their members, send out teachers to give them the latest techniques and advances in their field, and help establish spiritual centers where none existed before. Because of frequent border crossings and other cultural influences, the structure and the rituals of Mexican spiritual centers have had a strong influence on *curanderismo* in the United States. Spiritual centers now exist throughout Mexico, and the number in Mexican American and other Hispanic communities in the United States is steadily growing. These centers are spiritual churches called *templos* devoted to healing and communication with the dead. They have practicing mediums who counsel and heal, they train new mediums, and they have a regular calendar of events in which their members participate.

Certain activities are held on specific days of the week in these temples. One such temple set aside Tuesdays and Fridays for curing; Mondays, Wednesdays, and Thursdays were devoted to the *desarrollos* of new mediums and clairvoyants; on Saturdays sermons (*caceras*) were given explaining the scope, purpose, and philosophy of these centers; and Sundays were left free to allow people to go to mass or other church services. This temple also held occasional *dias de la luz* (days of light), during which malevolent spirits are invited to come down and possess mediums in the temples. Members of the temple would try to convert them from working in the bad or dark realm to working in the good or in the light.

There are many positions in these temples besides that of the medium. While the medium is working in trance, a clairvoyant (*vidente*) observes him. The *vidente* is a person who the *curanderos* say is capable of seeing into the spiritual world and reporting all that he has observed to the client. Each temple also has a rock, a guide, and columns. The rock is supposed to be a guardian of the temple and to protect the mediums from supernatural harm. If they are attacked by bad spirits, the rock is supposed to bring them out of trance and to protect them. One informant said, "He comes to be, symbolically, what Saint Peter represents in the Bible, guarding the gates of heaven." The guide gives the opening invocation and closing prayer for the spiritual session and is responsible for the smooth functioning of the temple. He decides on what days the cures or sermons will be held and how to schedule various activities in the temple. The columns stand in the temple and help the mediums if they have requests. They are the only members, except the guide, who are allowed to move around to any large extent during a spiritual session.

Once a temple has been established, it may have from one to twenty mediums working. The more mediums working, the better; otherwise, a medium may have to let his or her body be used by too many different spirits, which would exhaust the medium. The larger *templos* may have four or five *videntes*, as well as the mediums, and may be putting several apprentices through *desarrollo* at the same time.

Many Mexican Americans who believe in spiritualism (some coming from as far away as Illinois, California, and Oregon) travel into Mexico to visit the larger spiritual temples. The following is a description of one such temple given by a person who visited it regularly:

In Tampico [Mexico] there are several places where spiritualism is practiced with official permission. There is a spiritual association in Mexico that draws up a document that states that the persons in charge of such places have permission to help anyone who comes to see them. On various occasions I went to different temples and saw that this is something that people should know about. If you go to these places and ask for help, they don't demand any set amount of money; they ask you to give according to your means.

The persons who do the curing are dressed in white robes and they work in rooms adorned with blue and white, which is the symbol of the spiritual center. These persons are called mediums. A dead person's spirit is able to penetrate the medium, while he is in trance, and communicate with the people coming to the center.

In this center the patient enters the room where the medium is working and is swept with sweet basil (*albacar*) or with water prepared with lotion and ether. A *vidente* is also present to describe the spirit who comes to communicate through the medium and to identify some of the things associated with its visit to the client. The patient is allowed to speak with the spirits and either be healed or be given messages from the spirit world. The informant continued her description, saying:

One center is called Roca Blanca, because the spirit that predominates is called Roca Blanca. This center is about twenty-five years old. The owner's name is Lupita. She founded it after discovering she could cure after working in another center. She asked a spiritual association for permission to practice and it was granted.

I went to this place simply because I was curious. I was swept with *albacar* and the medium was at my side. While I was being swept, the medium went into trance. The sister who was sweeping me asked the spirit who he wanted to talk to. He said, "With the one you are sweeping." Then the sister finished sweeping me and directed me to talk with the person who was addressing me. When she [the medium in trance] talked to me, she sounded like a man. He asked me, "Do you know who I am?" I have a cousin who got killed in a place in Tampico. "You must be my cousin," I said. "Yes, exactly, I am your cousin." "Look," he said, "You have come here with your husband." On other occasions I really had been there with my husband, mother, and different relatives. "You have come here with your husband because you think he is hexed and that is why he is sick. But that's not true. He has a physical illness that the doctor can cure. Don't believe it's anything bad."

He said, "I'm going to prove who I am by coming to your house. Tell my cousin I'm going to see her." You see, I have a sister who's not nervous at all and who isn't afraid of anything. On Tuesday, as my sister was leaning by the window watching a television show, she felt someone embrace her. She turned and saw no one.

On another occasion, at three o'clock in the morning, I was awake and worried, because my husband was not home. I was afraid something had happened to him. So I asked that spirit, by name, to bring my husband home, whatever he was doing. At the moment I called the spirit, the rocker on the porch started rocking real fast, as if someone were in it. After a while it stopped. Ten minutes later my husband was home.

On another occasion we went to another center. As my mother went up front to get cured, he [the spirit of the informant's cousin] presented himself to her. He told her just because he was dead didn't mean he didn't do anything. He said everyone was assigned different work. Everyone had a job to work on. There were many spirits who wanted to communicate with this world, and he had presented himself because he had beaten the others to it.

They fight one another to come talk with persons they love or their relatives that are living. My mother asked him about my father, who is also dead; why didn't he present himself at these centers. The spirit said the reason was that "we're so many here that he doesn't have the chance to speak to anyone. Only ones who were mediums have the chance to come down."

From the evidence of these and other examples, the temples appear to serve a very important function beyond their attempts to cure various mental, physical, and spiritual disorders. They also help ease the pain and problems people have in relation to the death of members of their family. For these people the centers prove that there is a life after death and bring word of how the dead person's spirit is faring in his new existence.

Of course, not all of the centers are identical with the ones described above. They vary according to their size, the people developing them, and the spirits who associate with them. There are some people who believe they are complete fakery, others who believe they are evil, and some who are convinced that they produce miraculous cures and honest communication with the dead. It seems certain, regardless of the validity of any or all of these beliefs, that they serve an important social function within the communities in which they exist. They provide people with hope and counsel about physical, mental, and moral problems and they ease the problems of dealing with death.

The shamanism of the spiritual level should not be viewed in isolation, outside of its cultural context and function. Patients go to spiritual healers (wherever and however they practice) to get relief from physical, social, and spiritual problems. The ultimate goal of the spiritualists appears to be to provide relief through communication with the spiritual realm. This is achieved in much the same manner as on the material level of *curanderismo*: through counseling, through the administration of herbal baths, teas, and poultices, by means of changing positive and negative forces affecting the patient, by combating or reversing problems being created by spirits on the spiritual plane, and through magic. The major difference is that the agent bringing about the improved conditions is thought to be a spirit being working through the *curandero*, rather than the *curandero* himself.

On some occasions the spirits prescribe simple herbal remedies for physical problems of their patients. These recipes (*remedios*) are normally similar to the ones presented in the previous chapter, although occasionally a spirit will recommend a new use for an herb. These new remedies may then become common knowledge and continue to be used on the material level. On other occasions, the spirits may suggest that the patient perform the already familiar rituals of *curanderismo* (such as the *barrida*). As an example, an informant tells of a cure suggested by a medium in trance:

My brother-in-law was working at [a motel] in Weslaco. When he started working they laid off this other guy who had been working there for several years. This guy didn't like it, and he's been known to be messing around with black magic. I don't know what he did to my brother-in-law, but every other day he'd have to be taken home because he was sick. He started throwing up, had shaky knees and weak joints. So my mother and I went over to see this lady in Reynosa, and she told my mother just what to do. My sister rubbed her husband with a lemon every night for three days. She also gave him some kind of tea, but I don't remember what kind. On the third day a big black spot appeared on the lemon, so we threw it away and he's been fine ever since.

Spirits are also thought to be able to directly influence people's lives, in addition to having knowledge about material remedies. They control spiritual currents (*corrientes spirituales*) and mental vibrations (*vibraciones mentales*) that are capable of affecting the patient's health directly. Thus, spirits are thought to be able to manipulate the patient's fortune by directing positive or negative forces toward them from the spiritual realm. During spiritual sessions held at the developing center described earlier, a spirit repeatedly presented himself and treated several patients. One of these patients was a man in his early thirties who was suffering from lower back pains. One week he presented his back problem to the spirit and was told to buy an ace bandage and bring it to the next session. The man did so, but when he presented this bandage to the spirit the spirit chided him for not following his instructions correctly. The spirit said that the bandage was too narrow and not long enough. The man was instructed to buy a new bandage and place it on a window ledge to catch the morning dew (thought to have healing properties). Further, he was to place a glass of water under the head of his bed and a jar with alcohol at the side. He was to take the bandage, wrap himself with it as instructed, and lie quietly on his bed for no less than two hours, during which time the spirit promised to visit him and complete the cure. The man followed these instructions and said that he did gain relief from his back pain.

The same spirit treated a young college girl who periodically suffered asthma attacks. The girl's mother, a regular member of the group, brought her to the session when she was beginning to suffer an attack. The spirit stood and clasped her head with one hand on her *cerebro* and the other on her forehead, sending *corrientes espirituales* through her brain. The spirit then told her to take a sip of *agua preparada* and sit back down in the circle. This treatment was successful in overcoming this particular attack, and the mother mentioned that these cures often gave her relief for several weeks or months. When this evidence was presented to several physicians, they replied that such so-called cures were relatively common, because asthma and lower back pains often have psychological causes. The immediate results gotten from such cures rapidly reinforce the beliefs of the participants about the usefulness of these sessions.

Another patient asked this spirit for help for a social and emotional problem. Her husband had gotten into witchcraft (*brujeria*), and she was frightened that he or his friends might attack her or members of her family. A considerable amount of tension existed between the families, and she was under continual stress. She had been nervous for some time and had gone to a doctor for help. The doctor prescribed a mild sedative, which she had been taking for about three weeks without apparent relief. The spirit probed her mind, then told her to take three sips of *agua preparada* (presumably to break any spells against her). The spirit promised to provide her with protection and help from the spiritual realm, to counteract anything that her husband might do. She appeared to be content with the spirit's response.

Work on the spiritual level of *curanderismo* takes many forms. At its simplest it involves a single medium contacting the spiritual realm for cures and advice for patients. At its most complex it amounts to an organized religion existing in elaborate temple surroundings and serving hundreds, even thousands of persons daily.

The mediums who work on this level of *curanderismo* are shamans, and as such they represent the Mexican American cultural expression of a worldwide phenomenon. From the perspective of the participants in the system, mediums are able to establish communication with the spiritual realm. These links are used to comfort and to heal, as well as to irritate and to harm. Thus, spiritualism is becoming an important health resource in many Mexican American communities. It fits within the overall context of Mexican American folk medicine and is closely linked through symbols, rituals, and theories to the other levels of *curanderismo*.

Most of the cures that have been described above appear to have a strong psychosomatic element in them. This suggests that *curanderismo* has legitimate therapeutic value in this area and is responsible for alleviating the suffering of some patients with such problems. People also claim that it has therapeutic value for physical ailments, and they say they have witnessed cures of cancer, diabetes, and other physical problems. However, the research data compiled for this book neither substantiate nor refute this claim, since clinical studies of specific disease processes were not undertaken in conjunction with this particular project.

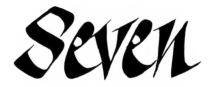

THE
MENTAL
LEVEL

THE MENTAL LEVEL (*nivel mental*) was the least commonly encountered of the three levels. The relative scarcity of this *don*, combined with the necessity for undergoing extensive training and rigorous discipline in order to practice on the mental level, greatly limits the number of healers who use those healing techniques.

The best way of detailing the activities of a *curandero* working on the mental level is to describe an encounter as a patient might see it and then provide the *curandero*'s perspective of the energies and processes they use. For the most part, the patient who is going to the *curandero* has no concept, or at best a vague idea, of how the *curandero* does his work. Most patients, according to the healers, expect something like a *barrida*, at least some kind of ritual performance. Consequently, many *curanderos* who work on the mental level add rituals to the healing process even though they are not felt to be necessary. Of the three levels, the mental level has the fewest rituals and the least complex visible behavior. It is not at all spectacular, although it is felt to be extremely effective.

The patient often begins an encounter with a healer by waiting. Some of the *curanderos* are extremely popular and may see twenty to sixty people each day. If the *curandero* practices in his home, the patient will normally wait in another room of the house, separate from the special room where the *curandero* practices but often within earshot of it. Sometimes the waiting room is a separate room, but most of the time it is merely a chair in one of the living rooms of the home, and as the patient waits to see the *curandero*, all of the normal household activities flow around and sometimes interact with the patient: children, pets, cooking, and friends. Some *curanderos* have offices or workrooms separate from their house (an older house, a trailer, or a garage), and there the waiting room is often a bench in the shade outside or a small room with old chairs or benches inside.

The patient is rarely alone. If the patient is a stranger to the *curandero*, he is normally accompanied by someone who does know the *curandero*. Even when the client is well known to the healer, it is common for another family member to accompany him. This is true even when the actual patient is not present. In that case two or more family members or friends will often approach the *curandero* to do healing at a distance. Although most of the informants said that they prefer for the client to come to them, and to come willingly, they all perform healing at a distance at the request of a concerned family member or friends. One of the reasons given for learning the mental level was to increase the healer's effectiveness in healing at a distance.

After a while the *curandero* will finish his current consultation and give that patient time to leave. Then the healer will either come to the door of the workroom and ask the waiting patient to enter, or simply call out for whoever is waiting to come in. We never observed very much interaction between patients leaving and those going in, beyond an occasional greeting. We do not know whether this was normal or simply peculiar to the situations we observed, but there was far less interaction between patients entering and leaving the healers' workrooms than we might have expected.

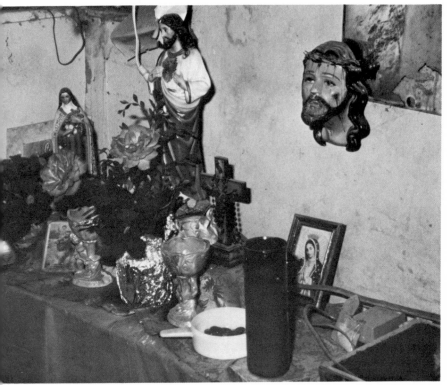

Altar in a *curandero*'s workroom

The patients enter the workroom and sit on chairs, couches, or benches. All of the workrooms had similar qualities, although each clearly reflected the personality and circumstances of the individual *curandero*. Each workroom contains an altar on a bench or table in the room. One or more crucifixes are displayed on the altar; sometimes one will be fixed to the wall above the table, with another lying on the table, handy for use in one of the *curandero*'s rituals. Several sorts of candles are often displayed on the altar, and one or more are normally lighted, especially if the healer works primarily on the material level. Some of the candles could be ordinary table candles in various colors. Other candles used are large and small votive candles. The large candles frequently have the drawing of a saint or the Virgin, along with a prayer and often a label or title telling what the candle is good for (good luck, house blessing, or tranquility, for example). These candles are produced commercially and sold in *boticas*, *yerberias*, and most grocery stores in the valley. The smaller votive candles may either be the plain kind sold in candle shops and most grocery stores, or they may have a paper covering depicting the Virgin of San Juan, who is very popular in the Lower Rio Grande Valley. Flowers are common on the altars. *Curanderos* working on the spiritual level are often requested by the spirits to keep specific varieties of flowers on their altar, because those flowers radiate beneficial vibrations for the spirits. Postcardlike drawings, paintings, and statues of saints and the Virgin are also an integral part of any healer's altar. The most popular saints on altars in the valley are San Martin de Porres (the Black Saint of Peru, who is noted for healing and helping the poor), San Martin Caballero (Saint Martin of Tours, also known for his work with the poor), San Antonio (Saint Anthony), and San Judas Tadeo (Saint Jude Thaddeus, patron saint of lost causes or impossible situations). The most popular virgin, by far, is the Virgin of San Juan de los Lagos. The Virgin of Guadalupe, who is so prominent in Mexico, is only occasionally found upon the healers' altars in the valley. This is partly due to the fact that there is a local shrine to the Virgin of San Juan, where many people go rather than going into Mexico to the original shrine. The local shrine has accrued enough miraculous events and a great enough reputation as a healing center to attract Mexican Americans from all over the United States and to make the Virgin of San Juan far more popular in the area than the Virgin of Guadalupe. The altars also contain objects from previous cures performed that day—eggs in glasses of water, burnt lemons, perfumes, and oils, to name a few. They may contain herbs or objects to be used in the cure for the next patient, if the healer knows in advance what will be needed for a particular cure.

The rest of the room also reflects the healer's vocation and personality. Many of the rooms we saw were painted bright blue or sky blue. This color is thought to aid in the healing and in mental exercises because it gives off vibrations that promote tranquility. One healer had an Egyptian bust in his workroom, a life-size plaster head of Nephratiti, because of some sort of connection with her which he said he was not allowed to discuss with us. Some *curanderos* have statues of the sitting Buddha in their offices, for good luck. One healer had a tropical fish aquarium with several types of fish in it and three bird cages with parakeets and canaries in them. When he was asked why, he said he simply liked them and liked having them in his office; they had no magical significance at all. Another healer had a composite photograph of the capitol in Washington, John F. Kennedy, and Abraham Lincoln. She said that Kennedy acted as a special protector of hers and that she kept the picture on her wall because of that. She and other *curanderos* also had purely decorative pictures and paintings on their walls.

When the patient is seated the *curandero* also sits, sometimes at a small desk or table, sometimes close to the table upon which the altar sits. These desks and small tables contain paraphernalia that the healers use in their consultations with patients. One of the most common items is a *copa* (a round bowl filled with water or sometimes empty and upside down, much like a crystal ball). When the *copa* is filled, it usually contains *agua preparada* (magically prepared water), which is used in various rituals. Sometimes the water is topped by a band of oil or perfume that has been chosen because of some magical properties that make the water more efficacious. The desk sometimes contains pads and pencils or pens that the healer uses to write down the patient's name and any information needed for the cure. This is done because some of the magical processes used in healing patients can only be performed at specific times, so the healer must keep track of what each patient needs and organize the work so that he does not either forget to do a particular cure at the proper time or forget which cure he had decided to use with a patient he saw hours or days ago.

Once the patient is sitting down, the next phase of interaction is much like any other personal social encounter: the participants sit and chat. After enough time has passed for confidence and rapport to be established, the healer gently steers the conversation in the direction of the problem that the patient has brought. The patient usually presents a general set of symptoms or complaints: insomnia, excessive drinking, misfortune in business, or marital troubles, for example. The *curandero* is then asked to pinpoint the cause of this disturbance and to remove it. To do so, the *curandero* goes through a diagnostic process to ascertain whether the cause is supernatural or natural and then to establish the exact cause and the best probable cure.

Diagnosis can be accomplished in many ways. Material-level techniques can be employed by the healer: reading cards for the patient, or sweeping the patient with eggs, candles, lemons, or other objects and then burning these objects. The cause and location of various ailments can be read from the shape and colors of the flames as the object burns or from the shape and color of various marks on the objects produced by the burning. One *curandera* gives *barridas* with eggs, cracks them in a glass of water, and then makes the diagnosis by reading the shapes of the white and shapes and colors on the yolk of the egg. On the spiritual level, the *curandero* can make the diagnosis, even at a distance, by sending his soul to look at the patient's soul or by asking spirits with whom the medium is in contact to check the patient. On the mental level, the *curandero* can make a diagnosis by observing the color, size, and shape of the patient's aura, or through mental readings or mental telepathy. Diagnosis on the mental level can also be done at a distance.

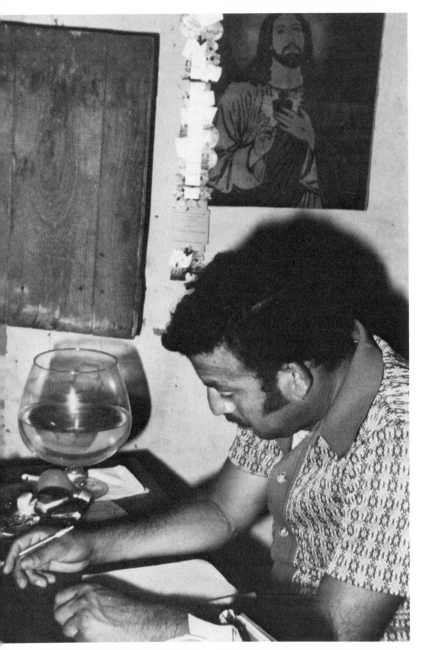

Curandero working on the mental level

The diagnosis can be done on any level the healer is capable of using, regardless of the level that is used in doing the cure. Thus, the diagnosis may be done on the material level and the cure on the mental level, or vice versa. The healer chooses a particular diagnostic technique according to the nature of the complaint and his or her own preferences and abilities. There are some limitations. For example, alcoholism can be treated by techniques of the mental and material systems but cannot be treated using the spiritual level (see Trotter and Chavira 1978). Therefore, the spiritual level is seldom used in the diagnosis of alcoholism.

To proceed with the therapy using the techniques of the mental level, the *curandero* asks the patient to state his complete name, if this has not been already asked during the diagnosis. Then the healer uses that name as a concentration point. From the patient's point of view the healer simply sits at the desk, staring at the paper upon which the patient's full name, and sometimes his birthday, is written. Then the healer closes his eyes and takes on a look of concentration. The healer stays in this attitude for a minute, five minutes, even longer. While this is going on the patient sits surrounded by near silence, hearing only the faint noises of the household and the neighborhood through the door and walls of the room. This appears to be an uncomfortable time for the clients, because so little seems to be happening. After the period of concentration the healer opens his eyes and begins talking with the patient. He tells the patient what he perceived while he was mentally searching the cause or root of the patient's problem. If the problem is magical, he may indicate who instigated the harm. Sometimes the culprit is described in a general way, sometimes minutely, and occasionally, we are told, an actual name is given. One of our informants made a point of never naming the sorcerer (*brujo*) who was causing the harm, only the person who had gone to that sorcerer. This, he said, protected the patients from themselves, since some had a tendency to want to confront not only their direct enemy, but also the *brujo*. He felt that doing so would lay them open for more harm than was already coming their way, especially if the *brujo* took offense.

After the *curandero* gives details about the patient's problem, he goes on to explain to the patient (or to the person who is asking help for someone else) that he has taken steps to overcome the problem, either by dominating the patient mentally to eliminate social and psychological problems or by channeling *vibraciones mentales* (mental vibrations) at the affected part of the patient's body, modifying its physical nature. After this, or at least as soon as the *curandero* feels that the patient is satisfied with what is happening, the *curandero* brings the session to a close and indicates whether the patient needs to return, and if so, how many more visits the cure will take. Patients are nearly always told their problems will be eliminated after a definite number of sessions (usually three, seven, or nine).

The healers themselves have a different perspective of the session. Their role is much more active than is outwardly visible. One informant says that he has learned through a developmental process (*desarrollo*) to use his mind as a transmitter, just as one would transmit waves from a radio station. He feels he can channel, focus, and direct *vibraciones mentales* at the patient. After asking if we understood the basic operation of a radio transmitter, the healer explained that he made the vibrations work in two ways: one physical, one behavioral. If he is working with a physical illness, such as cancer, then he channels the vibrations to the afflicted area, which he had previously pinpointed in the diagnosis, and uses the vibrations to retard the growth of the damaged cells and accelerate the growth of the normal cells around them. If the patient desires behavioral changes, he sends the vibrations into the person's mind and dominates it in a way that modifies the person's behavior. The *curandero* gave an example of one such case where the husband had begun drinking excessively, was unfaithful to his wife, was being a poor father to his children, and was in danger of losing his job. The *curandero* said that he dominated the man's thought processes and shifted them so the husband stopped drinking so much and became a model husband and father.

The developmental process for the mental level is different from that for the spiritual. Instead of a guided process, with considerable interaction with the healer during each lesson and even, according to the *curanderos*, direct magical manipulation by the teacher while the lesson is going on, the *desarrollo* for the mental level is one of personal exploration and discovery, often only minimally guided and explained by the teacher. The teacher does provide the student with exercises which must be mastered. Once an exercise is successfully performed, another is given, sometimes without explaining the usefulness of the earlier exercise. In fact, on the mental level the student is normally expected to figure out the meaning and wider ramifications of each exercise on his own.

The actual exercises used to instigate the *desarrollo* are quite numerous, but only three were provided to us. One exercise is to fill a clear smooth glass with water and hold it with the hands, thumbs on one side and fingers interlaced but flat on the glass on the other side. The palms of the hand do not touch the glass. The student then sits in a totally dark room and concentrates on "seeing" the glass and water. Partial success is achieved when he sees the rim of the glass as a bright blue line. More complete success means clearly seeing the glass and the water and, even better, also seeing millions of bright blue, infinitely small points of light flying out of the water. One informant described succeeding in this exercise:

> I was sitting on my couch holding this clear glass of
> water in my hands like P. [a healer] told me to. The room

was as dark as I could make it. After I had been sitting,
staring at the glass, for five minutes, I could just barely
see the glass in the gloom. Then an incredible thing happened. First, I saw the rim of the glass above the level of
the water. It was bright blue. Not sky blue or anything
like that, but a bright, neon-sign light blue, only much
purer in color. It was almost like a pure white light, that
kind of intensity, except it was bright blue instead of
white. If you haven't seen something like that then it is
very hard to describe, but once you've seen it and you
talk to someone else who's seen it, they understand what
you're talking about right away. After I watched that for
a while, I don't know how long, then I started seeing
these tiny blue sparks coming up out of the water. Millions of them, an infinite number of them. And they
were infinitely tiny. I don't know how to describe them.
They were so small that it was as if they weren't there,
yet the point of blue light made them visible. Thinking
back about it, they must look like what my high school
math teacher described as a true point, so small that it
has no dimensions but definitely exists. The word
chingos very aptly describes how many of these bright
blue points of light there were. The interesting thing was
that I could feel them, too. I was bending over the glass,
staring into it with my face six or eight inches away
from the rim. And these blue sparks flew up and hit my
face and I could feel them, at least some of them. They
didn't hurt; they tingled, something like the way the
bubbles from the fizz of Seven-up or the old fizzies
would feel. Ever since then, when I concentrate on water
I start feeling the tingling, even though I don't see the
blue sparks because I'm concentrating in the bathtub or
in a lighted room.

Another exercise is to place a mirror in front and then to
wipe one's own image from the mirror. However, the stu-

dent apparently does not see an empty mirror; the exercise is simply to achieve a blankness of vision even with one's eyes open. The mirror, according to one informant, is replaced by a dense gray fog or nothingness that indicates one has achieved the proper level of concentration. One informant who was still undergoing *desarrollo* said she had achieved the exercise of wiping her image off the mirror and that it had a profound effect on her. She said it was as if she had blanked out the self, leaving only an intellectual but unemotional observer. She said that as she achieved this level, a hole began to appear in the grayness that had replaced the mirror and she felt herself being drawn towards it. She began to be afraid, she lost concentration, and her image reappeared in the mirror. She had only succeeded in this exercise once, after weeks of trying, but she felt she had achieved a significant new step in her *desarrollo*, and that one day she would be able to step through the hole and see what was on the other side.

The third exercise was given to a student who was having difficulty getting results from the other two exercises. Not getting results is not uncommon at all. A person can apparently do an exercise every day for weeks or months with no result, suddenly achieve success, then be unable to repeat his success for a considerable length of time. The informants explained that these exercises are opening up new channels in the brain, and it takes time. This is one of the reasons the *curanderos* do not tell what will happen with the results; they merely tell how to do the exercise and instruct their pupils to report any results. Thus, they are able to check actual progress, rather than feigned progress. The third exercise that we collected was to sit in a darkened room and stare at a lighted candle. The focus of the apprentice's attention is the very point of the inner bluish flame that is surrounded by the more yellowish flame. The apprentice is to focus his total attention on that point, to the exclusion of everything else. Doing so is supposed to help his concentration so he can achieve the other exercises. We were never told what signaled that this exercise was successful, since the person performing it stopped the *desarrollo* process before it was completed.

The mental level and the spiritual level overlap somewhat in that the term *vibraciones mentales* is used in conjunction with both. However, on the mental level there is a reliance on the power available to the individual mind rather than on any relationship to spiritual entities. Also missing is any obvious tie to Christianity. None of the models of the Church were invoked to explain the mental level, although there was a tendency on the part of one informant to refer to the mental disciplines found in some of the Eastern religions, primarily Buddhism.

Beyond this limited information, the mental level simply awaits more thorough documentation, since we have concentrated our research on the other two areas. Practically all that can be currently verified is the basic explanatory model: the *curanderos* believe in a human ability to transmit and focus mental energies capable of modifying a person's physical or mental condition at a distance, and they can perform modifications in someone's condition with or without that person's knowledge.

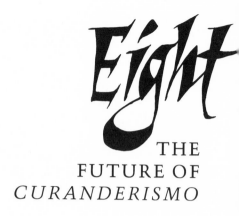

THE
FUTURE OF
CURANDERISMO

MOST OF THIS BOOK has dealt with the current status of the Mexican American folk-healing system in the Lower Rio Grande Valley of Texas. We have deliberately avoided bringing interpretive models other than the *curanderos'* own to bear on this ethnographic data. To have done so would have been to step outside the emic perspective of the healers, although such an approach is important for a social-science understanding of *curanderismo*. It is quite clear from our evidence that some inaccurate notions have been perpetuated in the scholarly literature. The biggest of these myths, for south Texas, is that *curanderismo* is dying out (see Crawford 1961, for example). It is not dying out; if anything, it is going through a period of considerable florescence and is gaining public respectability where it earlier had only private acceptance. The research efforts that produced the myth were undertaken at a time when many if not most social scientists contended that assimilation was the best possible alternative for Mexican Americans to take. The assumption, then, was that as Mexican Americans became more assimilated they would lose some of their traditional characteristics, such as their language and their belief in *curanderos*. Yet *curanderismo*, like the Mexican culture, continues to exist and to resist total assimilation because it satisfies basic psychological, spiritual, and health needs of the Mexican American communities. At the same time, there is no doubt that *curanderismo* is changing.

Curanderismo is changing because Mexican Americans are changing. They are undergoing cultural, educational, and occupational transformations that are bringing about new knowledge, new opportunities, different needs, and different ways of coping with social and environmental conditions. Also, the suspicion and distrust or avoidance of the medical care system reported by Rubel (1966) and Madsen (1960, 1964) has for all practical purposes disappeared in most of the Mexican American population. Since this negative attitude towards scientific medicine has, in the past, been seen as one element in the perpetuation of *curanderismo*, many of the interpretations of *curanderismo* need to be reexamined in light of the evidence that those attitudes have disappeared but *curanderismo* has not.

The isolation of the Mexican American, as far as health care is concerned, is fast dissolving. Educational levels are increasing for the population, and more education generally means better jobs and the ability to pay for private health care. Better jobs with large companies and both federal and state governments mean that health insurance is available for the worker and his or her dependents. The federal government has also done its share of making health care available to the indigent. Health clinics for migrant workers, well-baby clinics, immunizations, prenatal care, and school lunches are now important to the maintenance of health and the delivery of health services in the Lower Rio Grande Valley. This has caused some practices of *curanderismo* to disappear. For example, Madsen (1964) reports the existence of *hueseros* (persons who set broken bones) in south Texas in the late 1950s. There are no *hueseros* practicing today, since their function has been taken over by physicians, whose techniques have been proven superior to the old methods. By looking only for the practices that no longer exist, it might be possible to assume that *curanderismo* is dying out. Using the same logic, it might be assumed that medicine is dying out since there are no longer physicians who specialize in bleeding or using leeches. Evolution is not death.

One of the reasons for the continued existence of *curanderismo* is the *curandero*'s use of natural support systems, especially the family. For most Mexican Americans the social structure of illness and health is determined by the family system. Mexican American families have two salient characteristics: the majority are working-class families, and most are larger than the average American family. Most Mexican American, working-class families are child- and home-centered. These families revolve around the development and activities of their growing children, who are very important to the definition and function of the family system. This type of orientation gives a great deal of power and importance to the role of the woman and mother within the Mexican American family system. This importance is especially crucial in health care, since the woman must look after the sick and amass those resources necessary for successful rehabilitation. Therefore, the illness of a child or the illness of the mother can become a serious family problem from an emotional and a psychological point of view. The result of this home-family orientation is that illness may have greater relative social importance for Mexican Americans than for other ethnic groups.

For the marginally employed worker, stress, the likelihood of accidents, and the possibility of contamination (by insecticides, for example) make illness a constant threat. The lack of workman's compensation, sick leave, and family health insurance make it difficult for him and his family either to take time off to be sick or to pay for medical care. For some of these people, at least along the border, the *curandero* may actually become the only available health resource in the community, especially for those who fall between the cracks left by the various health services. To be among the nonmigrant poor of the valley is to have no reasonable access to health services that are not self-help services.

The *curanderos* provide a valuable counseling service for their clients, if absolutely nothing else. Their counsel includes all of the traditional types found within social work and psychology and tends to focus on courtship, marital, financial, legal, social, and business relationships. The healers use their knowledge of the client's personality and background, along with their own understanding of practical psychology, to provide him with counseling and advice which normally fit his own particular social, economic, and cultural needs. Health-care professionals have often been puzzled by the persistence of people's belief in magical causes of illnesses, despite clinically sound theories of the biological or psychological causation of disease. This persistence can be best explained by some of the social advantages that magical theories have over scientific theories.

Kiev (1968) is correct when he observes that the *curandero* is more a substitute for the psychiatrist than for the physician. Urbanization, technology, displacement, the installment plan, and the accessibility to medical care have modified the role of the *curandero*: he is now the main caretaker of mental hygiene in the *barrio*. The devastating emotional and psychological effects of modern living have possibly given *curanderismo* a more specialized meaning and a more specialized function than it previously had.

In order to explain the future prospects of *curanderismo*, as we see them, it is necessary to refer to some of the earlier works about the folk-healing system. The previous literature on *curanderismo* can be divided into two broad categories, descriptive and analytical. The descriptive articles and books range from simple cultural catalogs (for example, Curtin 1947; Holland 1963; Baca 1969), to detailed ethnographies (Clark 1959a; Madsen 1964; Sanders 1954; Rubel

1966). Each of these has certain limitations and all of them are now out of date for the valley, but some still provide worthwhile ethnographic details.

The major problem with the cultural-catalog articles is that they are lists of cultural traits that have been taken out of context and artificially presented in the literature. These articles are often compilations of remedies, descriptions of healing rites, or descriptions of objects used in specific rituals by folk healers. The emphasis is on show-and-tell descriptions, and the analysis of the data is normally superficial or nonexistent (Bourke 1894; Arnold 1928). These catalogs can be compared to butterfly collections. Butterflies mounted on the wall make pretty patterns and make butterflies attractive to look at, but these collections do not tell much about butterflies in the real world or how they live. The same can be said of the rituals or tools of folk healers when they are removed from their environment and displayed in articles or museums.

Researchers writing catalog articles have employed a variety of methodological approaches. Their major goal is, it seems, to answer the question, How can we best catalogue the different characteristics of *curanderismo* so that those characteristics make sense to us? Most of these articles interpret *curanderismo* in terms of scientific-professional logic which is not necessarily the logic employed by the practitioners and users of *curanderismo*. It is an attempt to give *curanderismo* the logical interpretation of the writer, not of the healer.

The writers of the ethnographic studies do not take anywhere near as simplistic approach to *curanderismo* as the cultural catalogs; however, most of the ethnographic accounts of Mexican American folk healing were produced as a byproduct of studies aimed at gathering other types of information. This all too often leads to generalizations and oversimplifications based on easily accessible information, but lacking in the richer details available from more fully documented, in-depth research focused on *curanderismo* it-self. But at least the information is normally placed within a described social and cultural context that makes *curan-derismo* a recognizable part of a total cultural system.

The interpretive articles are in a way both better and worse than the purely descriptive studies. Most researchers subscribe to a particular theoretical orientation—func-tionalism, neo-Marxism, conflict theory—and their re-search is colored, if not biased, by such an orientation. Yet most writers at least make the attempt to maintain some semblance of the social reality of the group they study in their presentations. Nevertheless, the interpretive studies tend to interpret the behavior they are describing purely from the logic of their explanatory paradigm. They do pro-vide explanations about behavior, and some of these expla-nations can even be tested by later research. Unfortunately, the information is often distorted into nearly unrecogniz-able form by the analysis. An example of both the good and the bad points of these analyses is the work by Ari Kiev (1968) in which he analyzes *curanderismo* from an un-abashedly Freudian analytical perspective. Where he sticks to description, the work appears to us to be compatible with our own, but in the analytical sections of the book, the cul-tural reality of the Mexican American community seems to become lost in Oedipal permutations.

Possibly the most common perspective used to analyze *cu-randerismo* is functionalism. Functional studies are works that analyze a subject in terms of the task or function that a cultural concept, belief, or behavior performs in maintain-ing social or psychological equilibrium for a group of people. Functional studies often emphasize role performance, social control, or social dysfunctions. Studies of role performance and social control show how the subject under investigation allows people to maintain a certain amount of smooth so-cial interaction because there are rules and sanctions for proper or against improper behavior. Some authors emphasize the negative by showing how dysfunctional behavior occurs or how it interrupts smooth interpersonal relationships. The articles that have a strongly psychological orientation point out the functions of certain types of behavior, usually to illustrate how such behavior acts to reduce stress or provide psychological support to a group of people caught in a psychologically disruptive situation.

People's belief in *curanderismo* has been described both as reinforcing Mexican American social values and cultural identification (Rubel 1960) and as providing a means for Mexican Americans to reject the pressures of acculturation to Anglo society (Clark 1959b:154–55). These are complementary but not identical functions. Another social function attributed to *curanderismo* is its usefulness in controlling people's behavior. The concept most often alluded to is the idea that since witchcraft (*brujeria*) is seen as dangerous, people will avoid antisocial behavior that might cause their neighbors to contract with a witch (*brujo*) to harm them. Thus, the existence of *brujeria* acts as a check on people's behavior.

The final social function that has been attributed to *curanderismo* is providing members of the community with rationalization for deviant behavior by producing socially acceptable explanations for socially unacceptable behavior or by providing a set of socially acceptable categories (statuses) for deviant individuals. The latter position states or suggests that some of the people who cannot adequately perform a normal role in society become *curanderos*, thereby making their inability to perform normal social roles acceptable, since no one could expect normal behavior of such an individual. However, the psychological or social abnormality of *curanderos* was in no way supported by the evidence we collected in numerous contacts with these people.

Psychologically oriented functional articles generally explain *curanderismo* from the perspective of the psychological functions the rituals perform for the community. These functions include the reduction of stress and mental disorders within the population (see Karno 1965; Kiev 1968; and Torrey 1972). Many scholars note that *curanderismo* is able to provide counseling or therapy within a social environment that is familiar and nonthreatening. Perhaps because mental health remains a frontier for modern medicine, the psychosomatic elements of *curanderismo* form the basis for its most avid support. Psychologists and psychiatrists have recognized the effectiveness of the *curandero* in dealing with various mental illnesses (see Kiev 1968; Kline 1969; Galvin 1961; and Torrey 1972) and suggest that *curanderos* or their healing techniques could be used to help Mexican American patients. Kiev's (1968:6) comments about *curanderismo* include the following: "It provides those with disorders such as chronic schizophrenia a kind of social support that enables them to continue to function in a supportive atmosphere. Thus, it serves prophylactic purposes. When these practices are no longer available, individuals who previously were able to cope are no longer able. *Curanderismo* is also important not only as a form of prevention which contributes to lower incidence but as a form of treatment agency whose presence leads to a reduced flow of people going to hospitals." Kline's (1969:94) suggestion is perhaps typical of those who want to incorporate *curanderos* into the mental-care system: "One way to deal with this community (Spanish American) resistance to treatment is to develop services with the participation of community leaders and traditional healers."

These observations and suggestions are valid from what is currently known about the cultural determinants of mental health, but a note of caution should be sounded before large-scale attempts are made to integrate *curanderos* into the medical system. As far as we can determine, no one has set up a situation in which psychiatrists or psychologists have intimately observed the patient-*curandero* interaction for any significant length of time. This seems analogous to diagnosing and suggesting treatment for a particular condition without having seen the patient's behavior. The diagnosis may be correct but should first be verified by empirical tests of the evidence. It seems unlikely that anyone should institute any new type of therapy system, and all of them have been new at one time, without first understanding exactly what the system entails.

Another problem is the difficulty of determining the *curanderos'* status within the health-care system. In their own communities, *curanderos* are the equivalent of the highest-ranking therapists. They determine both the cause and the cure of their patients' problems. Would they be accepted into the medical system on an equal status with the physician and clinical psychologist? Unlikely! They would probably be brought in as orderlies, assistants, or in some other low-status position. What would this do to their ability to treat the problem as they think it should be treated? How would they react to being under another therapist's orders? These questions must be seriously dealt with before the *curanderos* can be integrated into the conventional health-care system. There are others: the legal ramifications of practicing *curanderismo*, licensure, and criteria for selecting the correct *curandero* for a given position. Does the medical system need someone who heals on one, two, or all three levels of *curanderismo*? How is the establishment going to handle the supernatural concepts that exist on each level?

A few more questions need to be asked and answered before integrating *curanderos* into the system. Do the *curanderos* want to be made a part of the system? It may be that only second-rate *curanderos* or new and inexperienced ones would want to become a part of a clinic. The older, better, more experienced ones may have as much as they can handle at the present time, without being given additional patient loads by the establishment. As far as we can determine, no one has asked the healers if they want to join.

Another problem of working in a clinical setting is already recognized by the *curanderos*: the use of time and the place where therapy takes place. One healer says of the conventional system: "They limit themselves to treating the patient in the clinic only. They then have lots of problems because they just look at the subject they're treating without looking at their environment. They don't look at the family or whether they're having problems." The same healer went on to say that the clinics are often only open from eight to five, while he sees patients from early morning to nine or ten o'clock at night. Those hours suit him, since there is often free time in between patients, and they suit his clients, since they provide ready access to the healer. Could a clinic accommodate a system like this?

One final problem intrudes: the healing environment of *curanderismo*. We have been at some pains to provide detailed descriptions of both the physical and social environment within which *curanderismo* is practiced. The question becomes, What parts of this environment is it necessary to transfer to the clinic situation? Can those parts be transferred? Will they be compatible with or disruptive of other parts of the clinic situation? It is possible to envision a situation where a *curandero* is successfully installed in a clinic but profoundly disturbs patients who consider *curanderismo* a part of the devil's work on earth or who accept only "scientific truths" about reality. Many of these problems, and some others, are touched upon in the various articles in Velimirovic (1978).

Presenting these problems should not be taken to indicate that we oppose integrating *curanderos* into the medical system. If anything, we like the idea. But it would be unfortunate if such an attempt failed because no one took the experiment seriously enough to try to identify and eliminate the most pressing problems beforehand. The *curanderos* do have models for therapy that may be very useful to the conventional system. At least they have been successfully applied to some patients in their communities for significant periods of time, and they use the language, beliefs, and techniques of nonverbal communication that are most compatible with their patients' cultural framework. It has long been established that successful therapy for mentally ill patients depends heavily on the rapport between the therapist and the patient (Torrey 1972), and *curanderos* are past masters at developing and maintaining rapport with their clients.

The ability of most *curanderos* to use culturally and socially appropriate modes of therapy is very important, because human beings accept, reject, and modify their resources from within the total perspective of their social and cultural environment. Our research reveals that some families in south Texas actually have a family *curandero* as well as a family physician. It is not uncommon to find a family consulting both the *curandero* and the physician at the same time for the same illness. A case comes to mind which gives a good example of how the *curandero* and the physician can help each other as unseen colleagues.

Don José is an auto mechanic who underwent a gall-bladder operation at the age of seventy. After the operation he became depressed and continued to be depressed even after the doctor had said he was ready to go back to work. Don José believed the operation had made him weak and that he was sure to die. A few months after the operation, his wife called a *curandero* who came to see Don José at his house. After a series of three *barridas* to give him strength and spiritual energy, he went back to work. His depression was over, and he wanted to live. When asked what had the healer given him that the doctor had not, Don José answered, "*Animo!*" (enthusiasm). From this example, it is evident that some Mexican Americans make extensive use of modern health services, yet still have a definite need for the services of a *curandero*. To understand the tenacity of traditional health beliefs and practices one must view them not as dangerous or bizarre, but rather as of equal importance with other cultural traits such as language, food, and religion. The fact that Mexican Americans learn English and are exposed to hamburgers does not mean that they have to forget Spanish and stop eating tortillas. They learn to use English when it is appropriate and Spanish when it is appropriate. Cultural exposure generally expands resources and experiences, which is what happens to some patients who decide to use both modern medicine and *curanderismo*.

It has been shown over and over that the most important tool of the health-care provider is his or her ability to communicate with patients (Reusch and Bateson 1968). This ability becomes crucial in a social setting where the patient and the health-care provider have a different language and different cultural expectations. Some problems in communication will always exist between professionals and their patients. The concept of illness and treatment held by the professional is often remarkably different from the social framework of illness accepted by patients. It is also true that people can communicate best with others who share the same language, world views, and experiences. The greater the number of differences between the social frameworks of the healer and the patient, the more difficult communication becomes and the less likely it is that attempts at treatment will succeed. This communication factor complicates the problems of modern systems of health care because no two cultures, ethnic groups, social classes, or even professions share identical realities.

The extensive training given to all health-care professionals provides them with a social framework for illness that is different from that of nearly everyone else. Health-care professions share a common language about illness, a common understanding of the social roles of individuals in the health-care systems, and common experiences with illnesses. These common experiences make it much easier for professionals to communicate with each other than it is for them to communicate with their patients, who do not share their subculture of medicine. This extensive training—or socialization process—is necessary to allow professionals to cope with the complexity of human diseases and to acquire the technical skills needed to treat them. However, it is also this socialization process which forces practitioners to participate in a reality that is different from that of the people who seek their services. Normally there is enough overlap between the social reality of patient and practitioner to allow communication and understanding. However, it must be again emphasized that whenever the practitioner and the patient are members of different ethnic or cultural groups, communication may become difficult and sometimes impossible to achieve. In these cases, it is to the advantage of the health-care providers to seek exposure to the values and beliefs of their patients, if they wish to communicate with them.

We expect that *curanderismo*, because of its flexibility and adaptation, will continue to play an important role in the health status of Mexican Americans in the Lower Rio Grande Valley of Texas, especially in the area of mental health. As more persons become aware of *curanderismo*'s holistic approach to health, they may try to expand their demands for this approach from their physicians and their clergy as well. Especially relevant is the use of the whole family in the treatment of the sick, and the *curanderos'* awareness of the long-range social and psychological effects of illness. *Curanderismo* can be taken as a model of a health system that incorporates concepts from the social and behavioral sciences in its therapeutic regimens. Perhaps this trait is what makes *curanderismo* appear to us to be such a vital health resource: it combines self-reliance with cultural relevance and family systems and gives some Mexican Americans a sense of stability and continuity in the face of socially disrupting urban-technological change. It provides a linkage of past and future in a therapeutic system.

It is clear to us, from the data we have presented, that all future research into *curanderismo* must take into account

its systemic nature. Treating it as a mass-cultural phenomenon, as has been done in the past, may be valuable for showing the depth and spread of what can be considered technical
knowledge throughout the culture, just as similar studies
on the spread of technical information from medical systems are valuable. But to ignore the systemic attributes of
curanderismo would be to apply an incorrect analysis to the
subject by ignoring its theoretical components. Another
matter for further research is the energy concept that appears to be the central idea unifying the three levels of *curanderismo*. Another area of interest might be the Christian
symbols and theology which act as additional organiza-
tional models for both the material level and the spiritual
level, but not for the mental level. The spiritual and mental
levels are both in a state of transition in the Lower Rio
Grande Valley, and it will take some time for them to become more stable, less idiosyncratic. The spiritual temples
now being established will have a considerable stabilizing
effect on spiritualism there. However, the mental level is
likely to remain far more idiosyncratic in its application
than the other levels, not only because of its newness but
also because the gift requires a very different developmental
process (*desarrollo*). In all, *curanderismo* is active in the
Lower Rio Grande Valley of Texas, and it appears that it will
remain so. It should be worthy of study for years to come.

APPENDIX

Las Doce Verdades del Mundo

De las doce verdades del mundo, decidme una,
 La santa casa de Jerusalén.
De las doce verdades del mundo, decidme dos,
 Las dos tablas de Moisés.
De las doce verdades del mundo, decidme tres,
 La santa Trinidad.
De las doce verdades del mundo, decidme cuatro,
 Los cuatro evangelios.
De las doce verdades del mundo, decidme cinco,
 Las cinco llagas.
De las doce verdades del mundo, decidme seis,
 Los seis candelabros.
De las doceverdades del mundo, decidme siete,
 Las siete palabras.
De las doce verdades del mundo, decidme ocho,
 Las ocho angustias.
De las doce verdades del mundo, decidme nueve,
 Los nueve meses de María.
De las doce verdades del mundo, decidme diez,
 Los diez mandamientos.
De las doce verdades del mundo, decidme once,
 Las once mil vírgenes.

De las doce verdades del mundo, decidme doce,
    Las doce apóstoles que acompanaron a
    nuestro Señor en la cruz.

                      Amén

The Twelve Truths of the World

Of the twelve truths of the world, tell me one,
    The holy house of Jerusalem.
Of the twelve truths of the world, tell me two,
    The two tablets of Moses.
Of the twelve truths of the world, tell me three,
    The Holy Trinity.
Of the twelve truths of the world, tell me four,
    The four evangelists.
Of the twelve truths of the world, tell me five,
    The five wounds.
Of the twelve truths of the world, tell me six,
    The six candelabras.
Of the twelve truths of the world, tell me seven,
    The seven words.
Of the twelve truths of the world, tell me eight,
    The eight anguishes.
Of the twelve truths of the world, tell me nine,
    The nine months of Mary.
Of the twelve truths of the world, tell me ten,
    The Ten Commandments.
Of the twelve truths of the world, tell me eleven,
    The eleven thousand virgins.
Of the twelve truths of the world, tell me twelve,
    The twelve apostles who accompanied
    our Lord on the cross.

                      Amen

GLOSSARY

Aceite de las siete potencias. Oil of the seven African potencies; sold in yerberias and often used in ritual baths.

Aceite de vibora. Rattlesnake oil; in this study, used to keep people from gossiping.

Aceite preparado. Oil especially prepared to cut the negative currents and vibrations which surround the patient.

Agua preparada. Water especially prepared to enhance its spiritual potential.

Albacar. Sweet basil (*Ocimum basilicum*).

Animas. Spirits; souls.

Ánimo. Enthusiasm.

Anis. Anise (*Pimpinella anisum*).

Auras. Bands of energy or light that can be perceived outlining an individual; they are sometimes used to diagnose illnesses.

Barrida. A spiritual sweeping designed to bring about relief of a physical, emotional, or spiritual discomfort.

Barrio. Mexican American neighborhood.

Bilis. Folk illness brought about by excessive and prolonged anger and fear; manifests itself as a stomach disorder.

Borraja. Borage (*Borago officinalis*).

Botica. Drugstore; in this study, synonymous with *yerberia*.

Brujeria. Witchcraft.

Brujo or *bruja.* Sorcerer or witch; works evil spells.

Cáscara sagrada. Cascara sagrada (*Rhamnus californica*).

Cátedra. Sermons and instructions given to members of spiritualist centers on specific days.

Centros. Spiritualist centers staffed by trance mediums.

Centros espiritistas. See *centros.*

Cerebro. Cerebellum.

Cerebro debil. A weak cerebellum, which cannot communicate with the spiritual realm.

Ciencias ocultas. Occult sciences.

Conjuros. Conjures.

Copa. A bowl of water (*agua preparada*) always present in a *curandero's* office.

Copal. Copal, used in the incense for some *sahumerios.*

Corrientes espirituales. Spiritual forces which can be used to cause, diagnose, or cure an illness.

Corrientes mentales. Psychic energy or mental currents.

Curación. A complete ritual which may involve a *barrida,* prayers, baths, diet, and so forth, designed to eliminate a special problem.

Curanderismo. The Mexican American folk-healing system.

Curandero. A Mexican American folk healer.

Curioso. Peculiar; odd; strange.

Desarrollo. Development of healing potential at the spiritual and mental levels.

Dias de la luz. Literally, days of light; special days dedicated to convincing malevolent spirits to become good.

Don Pedrito Jaramillo. A famous healer from Los Olmos, Texas.

El daño. Literally, the harm; may mean the actual illness or its representation, for example, candles, dolls, or other objects.

El don. The gift of healing.

Envidia. Envy or resentment; sometimes taken to be the cause of ill will and sorcery against a patient.

Espiritistas. Spiritualist mediums; sometimes used synonymously with *espiritualistas.*

Espiritualistas. Spiritualists; trance mediums; sometimes used synonymously with *espiritistas.*

Espíritu malo. Evil spirit.

Espiritus. Spirits; souls.

Espiritus de luz. Benevolent spirits.

Espiritus obscuros. Evil spirits.

Estilos de helote or *pelos de helote.* Corn silk (*Zea mays*).

Estoraque. An incense used for *sahumerios.*

Fidencistas. Followers of el Niño Fidencio.

Flor de tila. Linden flower (*Tiliaceae europaea* Linn.).

Fresno. Ash tree (*Fraxinus* sp.).

Haba marina. Unidentified medicinal plant.

Habas de San Ignacio. Seed of the monkey dinner bell tree (*Hura polyandra* L. or *Hura crepitans* L.)

Hermano guardian. Protector of the spiritualist temple.

Huachachile. *Loscelia scariosa* Mart. et Gal.

Hueseros. Healers who specialize in setting broken bones and treating joint injuries.

La cachana y el cachano. Unidentified medicinal plant.

La frente. The forehead.

Las Doce Verdades del Mundo. Prayer recited in sweepings.

La Virgen de Guadalupe. Our Lady of Guadalupe; the official patron of Mexico and a major symbol of national pride and cultural identity.

La Virgen de San Juan. Our Lady of San Juan; believed by many to be the unofficial patron of Mexican Americans, especially migrant farm workers; venerated at her shrine and major healing center in San Juan, Texas.

Limpia. A ritual sweeping designed to protect a person from harm, to remove bad influences, and to provide spiritual strength.

Linaza. Linseed (*Linum usitatissimum*).

Lo bueno. The good.

Lo malo. The evil.

Mal puesto. A hex which causes misfortune or illness.

Malva. Malva; cheeseplant (*Malva neglecta*).

Manzanilla. Camomile (*Matricaria chamomilla*).

Mesaje. Massage for aches due to nervous tensions.

Medium. A person capable of allowing a spirit to possess his or her body and use it to communicate with a patient.

Mejorania. Marjoram (*Origanuum onites*).

Myrrha. Myrrh, used as an incense in *sahumerios*.

Niño Fidencio. A famous *curandero* from Espinaso, Mexico.

Nivel espiritual. Spiritual level; involves the intercession and manipulation of spiritual beings.

Nivel material. Material level; involves the manipulation of material objects and symbols, for example, candles and herbs.

Nivel mental. Mental level; involves the ability to transfer and manipulate psychic energy.

Nopal. Prickly pear cactus (*Opuntia ficus-indica*).

Oregano. Oregano (*Oreganum valagare* L.).

Partera. Midwife.

Peyote. Peyote (*Lophophora williamsii*).

Piedra alumbre. Alum.

Plática. Conversation.

Propiedades magnéticas. Magnetic properties; give strength to *agua preparada* and *aceite preparado*.

Remedios caseros. Home remedies.

Romero. Rosemary (*Rosmarinus officialis*).

Rosa de Castilla. Rose petals (*Rosa* sp.).

Ruda. Rue (*Ruta graveolens*).

Sahumerio. Ritual incensing which is strictly a purification rite.

Salaciones. Bad luck or disharmony manifested by business failure, marital disruption, unemployment, delinquency, or other social pathology.

San Antonio de Padua. St. Anthony of Padua; a favorite intermediary for all kinds of requests. It is widely believed that in order to get St. Anthony to listen, he must be turned upside down until the request is granted.

San Judas Tadeo. St. Jude Thaddeus; one of the Twelve Apostles, universally known as the patron saint of the impossible or lost causes.

San Martin Caballero. St. Martin of Tours; Roman centurion who gave his cloak to a beggar.

San Martin de Porres. St. Martin de Porres; the black Peruvian saint who has attracted considerable following in the last fifteen years. He is famous for healing and helping the poor.

San Miguel Arcangel. St. Michael the Archangel. In spiritual centers, St. Michael often acts as a spiritual protector to ward off evil spirits which may interfere with a session.

Sobadita. Treatment for specific muscle problems.

Sobadores. Persons who massage muscle aches and pains usually caused by work, exercise, or chronic conditions; occupational therapists.

Sortilegio. Conjure designed to influence the life of the petitioner by removing obstacles in his daily life.

Templos. Spiritualist centers or spiritualist temples.

Tendidas. The different stages involved in card readings.

Trabajo. A spell or a magical act.

Trabajo negro. An act which promotes evil and illness.

Velaciones. A candling ritual intended to influence people from a distance.

Verbena. Vervain (*Verbena macdougalii*).

Vidente. A person with the ability to predict the future; a clairvoyant.

Vibraciones. Vibrating energy present in all persons, animals, and certain material objects.

Vibraciones mentales. Psychic energy.

Yerba buena. Spearmint (*Mentha spicata*).

Yerba de la golondrina. May be *Euphorbia prostrata*.

Yerba del coyote. Coyote weed (*Polanisia uniglandulosa* Cav.).

Yerba del cusito. Jamaica mountain sage (*Lantana camara* L.).

Yerba del gato. Catmint, catnip (*Nepeta cateria*).

Yerba del pájaro. Unidentified medicinal plant.

Yerba de San Nicolas. *Tecoma mollis* H.B.K.

Yerba del trueno. Unidentified medicinal plant.

Yerberia. Herb shop; also stocks candles, incense, religious articles, oils, perfumes, and other products used by *curanderos* and their patients.

Yerberos or *yerberas.* Persons knowledgeable about herbal remedies.

REFERENCES

Aguirre, Lydia
   1978   Alternative Health Practices along the Western Texas
          Border. *In* Modern Medicine and Medical Anthropology
          in the United States–Mexico Border Population. Boris
          Velimirovic, ed. Washington, D.C.: Pan American Health
          Organization. Scientific Publication no. 359.

Alegria, Daniel, Ernesto Guerra and Cervando Martinez, Jr.
   n.d.   El Hospital Invisible: A Study of Curanderos. Mimeo-
          graph. Department of Psychiatry, University of Texas
          Health Science Center at San Antonio.

Alger, Norman
   1974   The Curandero-Supremo. *In* Many Answers. Norman Al-
          ger, ed. New York: West Publishing.

Alvarado, Anita L.
   1978   Utilization of Ethnomedical Practitioners and Concepts
          within the Framework of Western Medicine. *In* Mod-
          ern Medicine and Medical Anthropology in the United
          States–Mexico Border Population. Boris Velimirovic, ed.
          Washington, D.C.: Pan American Health Organization.
          Scientific Publication no. 359.

Arias, Hipólito y Felix Costas
   n.d.   Plantas medicinales. Mexico: Biblioteca Practica.

Arnold, Charles A.
   1928   The Folklore, Manners, and Customs of Mexicans in San
          Antonio, Texas. M.A. thesis, University of Texas.

Baca, Josephine
  1969   Some Health Beliefs of the Spanish Speaking. American
         Journal of Nursing 69:2171–2176.
Bard, Cephas L.
  1930   Medicine and Surgery among the First Californians.
         Touring Topics.
Bluestone, H. R.
  1969   The Establishment of a Mental Health Service in a Pre-
         dominantly Spanish-speaking Neighborhood of New
         York City. Behavioral Neuropsychiatry 5:12–16.
Boatright, Mody C., Wilson M. Hudson, and Allen Maxwell, eds.
  1954   Texas Folk and Folklore. Dallas: Southern Methodist
         University Press.
Bourke, John H.
  1894   Popular Medicine Customs and Superstitions of the Rio
         Grande. Journal of American Folklore 7:119–146.
Brooks County Historical Survey Committee
  1972   Don Pedrito Jaramillo: 1829–1907: The Faith Healer of
         Los Olmos. Falfurrias, Tex.: Brooks County Historical
         Society.
Buckland, Raymond
  1970   Practical Candle Burning. St. Paul, Minn.: Llewellyn Pub-
         lications.
Capo, N.
  n.d.   Mis observaciones clinicas sobre el limon, el ajo, y la
         cebolla. Mexico, D.F.: Ediciones Natura.
Cheney, Charles C., and George L. Adams
  1978   Lay Healing and Mental Health in the Mexican Ameri-
         can Barrio. In Modern Medicine and Medical Anthropol-
         ogy in the United States–Mexico Border Population.
         Boris Velimirovic, ed. Washington, D.C.: Pan American
         Health Organization. Scientific Publication no. 359.
Clark, Margaret
  1959a Health in the Mexican American Culture. Berkeley: Uni-
         versity of California Press.
  1959b Social Functions of Mexican American Medical Beliefs.
         California's Health 16:153–155.
Comas, Juan
  1954   Influencia indígena en la medicina Hipocrática en la

Nueva España del siglo XVI. Americana Indigena 14(4): 327–361. Mexico, D.F.

Cosminsky, Sheila
  1978   Midwifery and Medical Anthropology. *In* Modern Medicine and Medical Anthropology in the United States–Mexico Border Population. Boris Velimirovic, ed. Washington, D.C.: Pan American Health Organization. Scientific Publication no. 359.

Crawford, Fred R.
  1961   The Forgotten Egg. Austin: Texas State Department of Public Health.

Creson, D. L.
  1967   An Interview with a Curandero. Paper presented to the 8th Annual Titus Harris Society Meeting.

Creson, D. L., C. McKinley, and R. Evans
  1969   Folk Medicine in Mexican American Subculture. Diseases of the Nervous System 30:264–266.

Currier, R. L.
  1966   The Hot-Cold Syndrome and Symbolic Balance in Mexican and Spanish American Folk Medicine. Ethnology 4:251–263.

Curtin, L. S. M.
  1947   Healing Herbs of the Upper Rio Grande. Santa Fe: Laboratory of Anthropology.

Davis, Jacaleen
  1979   Witchcraft and Superstitions of Torrance County. New Mexico Historical Review 54:53–58.

Dodson, Ruth
  1932   Folk Curing among the Mexicans. *In* Tome the Bell Easy. Texas Folklore Society. Dallas: Southern Methodist University Press.
  1954   Curandero of Los Olmos. *In* Texas Folk and Folklore. Boatright et al., eds. Dallas: Southern Methodist University Press.
  1972   Folk Curing among the Mexicans. *In* Cultural Differences in Medical Care. Robert H. Gemmill, ed. pp. 59–76. Ft. Sam Houston, Tex.: Academy of Health Sciences, United States Army.

Edgerton, R. B., M. Karno, and I. Fernandez
  1970   Curanderismo in the Metropolis: The Diminished Role

of Folk Psychiatry among Los Angeles Mexican Americans. American Journal of Psychiatry 24:124–134.

Esteyneffer, Juan de, S. J.

1711   Florilegio medicinal de todas las enfermedades, sacado de varios, y clasicos autores, para bien de los pobres y de los que tienen falta de medicos en particular para las provincias remotas en donde administran los RR.PP. Mexico: Misioneros de la Compania de Jesus. Microfilm.

1887   Florilegio medicinal o breve epidome de las medicinas y cirujia. Mexico. First ed. 1713.

Evans-Pritchard, E. E.

1937   The Notion of Witchcraft Explains Unfortunate Events. In Witchcraft, Oracles, and Magic among the Azande. Oxford: Oxford University Press.

Fabrega, Horacio, Jr.

1970   On the Specificity of Folk Illness. Southwestern Journal of Anthropology 26:305–315.

1973   Illness and Shamamatic Medicine among the Zinancantarones. Stanford, Calif.: Stanford University Press.

Fantini, Albino

1962   Illness and Curing among the Mexican Americans of Mission, Texas. M.A. thesis, University of Texas.

Farfán, Agustín.

1944   Tractado breve de medicina. First ed. Mexico: Pedro Ocharte, 1592. Reprint. Colección de Incinables Americanos, vol. 10. Madrid: Ediciónes Cultura Hispanica.

Farge, E. J.

1977   Review of Findings from Three Generations of Chicano Health Care Behavior. Social Science Quarterly 58:407–411.

Foster, G. M.

1953   Relationships between Spanish and Spanish American Folk Medicine. Journal of American Folklore 66:201–247.

Frazer, James G.

1922   The Golden Bough. New York: Macmillan.

Friedson, Elliot

1970   Professional Dominance: The Social Structure of Medical Care. Chicago: Aldine.

Galvin, James A. V., and Arnold M. Ludwig

1961   A Case of Witchcraft. Journal of Nervous and Mental Disease. pp. 161–168.

Garcia, R. L.
1977   "Witch Doctor?" A Hexing Case of Dermatitis. Cutis 19(1): 103–105.

Gillin, J.
1948   Magical Fright. Psychiatry 11: 387–400.

Givry, Grillot de
1971   Witchcraft, Magic, and Alchemy. Courtenay Locke, trans. New York: Dover.

Gobeil, O.
1973   El Susto: A Descriptive Analysis. International Journal of Social Psychiatry 19: 38–43.

Gudeman, Stephen
1976   Saint, Symbols, and Ceremonies. American Ethnologist 3(4): 709–730.

Guerra, Francisco
1961   Monardes. Dialogo de Hierro. N.p.: Companiá Fundido de Fierro y Acero de Monterrey.
n.d.   Los cronistas hispanoamericanos de la materia medicina colonial. *In* Homenaje ofrecido al Profesor Dr. Teofilo Hernando por sus amigos y discipulos. Madrid: Libreria y Casa Editorial Hernando.

Hamburger, S.
1978   Profile of Curanderos: A Study of Mexican Folk Practitioners. International Journal of Social Psychiatry 24: 19–25.

Hanson, Robert C., and Mary J. Beach
1963   Communicating Health Arguments across Cultures. Nursing Research 12: Fall.

Hanson, Robert C., and Lyle Saunders.
1964   Nurse–Patient Communication: A Manual for Public Health Nurses in New Mexico. Santa Fe: The New Mexico State Department of Public Health.

Harner, Michael J.
1973   Hallucinogens and Shamanism. New York: Oxford University Press.

Hoebel, E. A.
1972   Anthropology: The Study of Man, 4th ed. New York: McGraw-Hill.

Holland, W. R.
  1963   Mexican-American Medical Beliefs: Science or Magic? Arizona Medicine 20:89–102.

Hudson, Wilson M.
  1951   The Healer of Los Olmos and Other Mexican Lore. Austin, Tex.: Texas Folklore Society 24.

Huson, Paul
  1970   Mastering Witchcraft: A Practical Guide for Witches, Warlocks, and Covens. New York: G. P. Putnam's Sons.

Ingham, J. M.
  1940   On Mexican Folk Medicine. American Anthropologist 42:76–87.

Jaco, E. Gartley
  1957   Social Factors in Mental Disorders in Texas. Social Problems 4(4):322–328.
  1959   Mental Health of the Spanish-American in Texas. In Culture and Mental Health. Marvin K. Upler, ed. New York: Macmillan.

Johnson, C. A.
  1964   Nursing and Mexican-American Folk Medicine. Nursing Forum 3(2):100–112.

Kardec, Allan
  1970   Book on Mediums. New York: Samuel Weiser.

Karno, Marvin.
  1966   The Enigma of Ethnicity in a Psychiatric Clinic. Archives of General Psychiatry 14:516–520.
  1969   Mental Health Roles of Physicians in a Mexican-American Community. Community Mental Health Journal 5(1).

Karno, Marvin, and Robert B. Edgerton
  1969   Perception of Mental Illness in a Mexican-American Community. Archives of General Psychiatry 20:233–238.

Kay, Margarita
  1972   Health and Illness in the Barrio: Women's Point of View. Ph.D. dissertation, University of Arizona.
  1974a The Fusion of Utoaztecan and European Ethnogynecology in the Florilegio Medicinal. Paper presented at Medical Anthropology Symposium, 41st International Congress of Americanists, Mexico City. Publication forthcoming: Proceedings 41st International Congress of Americanists.

1974b   Florilegio Medicinal: Source of Southwestern Ethno-medicine. Paper presented to the Society for Applied Anthropology, Boston.

1978   Parallel, Alternative, or Collaborative: Curanderismo in Tucson, Arizona. *In* Modern Medicine and Medical Anthropology in the United States–Mexico Border Population. Boris Velimirovic, ed. Washington, D.C.: Pan American Health Organization. Scientific Publication no. 359.

Kearney, Michael

1978   Espiritualismo as an Alternative Medical Tradition in the Border Area. *In* Modern Medicine and Medical Anthropology in the United States–Mexico Border Population. Boris Velimirovic, ed. Washington, D.C.: Pan American Health Organization. Scientific publication no. 359.

Kelley, Isabel

1965   Folk Practices in North Mexico. Austin: University of Texas Press.

Kiev, Ari

1968   Curanderismo: Mexican American Folk Psychiatry. New York: Free Press.

Kieve, Rudolph

1961   The Meaning and Use of Illness and Disability Among Spanish-speaking People in Northern New Mexico. Presented at the 4th Western Divisional Meeting of the American Psychiatric Association, 21 September 1961, in Salt Lake City.

Kimber, Clarissa

1973   Plants in the Folk Medicine of the Texas-Mexico Borderlands. Proceedings of the Association of American Geographers, pp. 130–133.

1974   Curing Mediums and Medicinal Plants in the Valley of Texas. Paper presented at the 73rd Annual Meeting of the American Anthropological Association.

Klein, Janice

1978   Susto: The Anthropological Study of Diseases of Adaptation. Social Science and Medicine 12:23–28.

Kleinman, Arthur

1978   Culture, Illness, and Care: Clinical Lessons from Anthropologic Cross-Cultural Research. Annals of Internal Medicine 88:251–258.

Kline, L. Y.
    1969   Some Factors in the Psychiatric Treatment of Spanish-Americans. American Journal of Psychiatry 125:1674–1681.

Kreisman, Jerold J.
    1975   Curandero's Apprentice: A Therapeutic Integration of Folk and Medical Healing. American Journal of Psychology 132(1):81–83.

Langner, T. S.
    1965   Psychophysiological Symptoms and the Status of Women in Two Mexican Communities. Approaches to Cross-Cultural Psychiatry. Ithaca, N.Y.: Cornell University Press, pp. 360–392.

Lawrence, Trinidad Flores Limon, Louis Bozetti, and Terry J. Kane
    1976   Curanderos: A Unique Role for Mexican Women. Psychiatric Annals 6(1).

Macklin, June
    1962   The Curandera and Structural Stability in Mexican-American Culture: A Case Study. A paper presented to the American Anthropological Association, Chicago.
    1965   Current Research Projects. Curanderismo among Mexicans and Mexican Americans. New London: Connecticut College.
    1967   El Niño Fidencio: Un estudio del curanderismo en Nuevo Leon. Anuario Humánitas. Centro de Estudios Humanisticos. University of Nuevo Leon.
    1974a   Santos folk, curanderismo, y cultos espiritistas en Mexico: Elección divina y selección social. Anuario Indigenista 34:195–214.
    1974b   Folk Saints, Healers and Spiritist Cults in Northern Mexico. Revista Interamericana 3(4):351–367.
    1974   Belief, Ritual, and Healing: New England Spiritism Compared. In Religoius Movements in Contemporary America. I. Zaretsky and M. Leone, eds. pp. 383–417. Princeton: Princeton University Press.
    1978   Curanderismo and Espiritismo: Complementary Approaches to Traditional Mental Health Services. In Modern Medicine and Medical Anthropology in the United States–Mexico Border Population. Boris Velimirovic, ed. Washington, D.C.: Pan American Health Organization. Scientific Publication no. 359.

Macklin, June, and N. Ross Crumring
  1973   Three North Mexican Folk Saint Movements. Compara-
         tive Studies in Society and History 15(1):89–105.

Madsen, Claudia
  1965   A Study of Change in Mexican Folk Medicine. Middle
         American Research Institute 25:93–134.

Madsen, William
  1955a Shamanism in Mexico. Southwestern Journal of An-
         thropology 2:48–57.
  1955b Hot and Cold in the Universe of San Francisco Tecospa,
         Valley of Mexico. Journal of American Folklore, pp.
         123–139.
  1961   Society and Health in the Lower Rio Grande Valley. Aus-
         tin, Tex.: Hogg Foundation for Mental Health.
  1964a The Mexican Americans of South Texas. New York:
         Holt, Rinehart, and Winston.
  1964b Value Conflicts and Folk Psychotherapy. In Magic, Faith
         and Healing. Ari Kiev, ed. pp. 420–444. New York: Free
         Press.
  1966   Anxiety and Witchcraft in Mexican-American Accultura-
         tion. Anthropology Quarterly, pp. 110–127.

Mair, Lucy
  1969   Witchcraft. New York: McGraw-Hill.

Malinowski, Bronislaw
  1935   Coral Gardens and Their Magic. 2 vols. London: George
         Allen and Unwin.
  1948   Magic, Science, and Religion. In Magic, Science, and Re-
         ligion and Other Essays. Boston: Beacon Press.

Marcos, Luis R., and Murry Alpert
  1976   Strategies and Risks in Psychotherapy with Bilingual Pa-
         tients. American Journal of Psychiatry 113(11):1275–
         1278.

Martinez, Cervando, and Harry W. Martin
  1966   Folk Diseases among Urban Mexican Americans. Journal
         of American Medical Association 196:161–164.

Maus, Marcel
  1972   A General Theory of Magic. New York: W. W. Norton.

McFeely, F.
  1956   Some Aspects of Folk Healing in the American South-
         west. Anthropological Quarterly 29:95–110.

Montiel, Miguel
    1970   The Social Science Myth of the Mexican American Family. El Grito 3:4.

Morales, Armand
    1970   Mental Health and Public Health Issues: The Case of the Mexican Americans in Los Angeles. El Grito 3(2).

Moustafa, A. Taher, and Gertrude Weiss
    1968   Health Status and Practices of Mexican Americans. Graduate School of Business, University of California.

Moya, Benjamin
    1940   Superstitions and Beliefs among the Spanish Speaking People of New Mexico. M.A. thesis, University of New Mexico.

Nall, Frank C., and Joseph Speilberg
    1967   Social and Cultural Factors in the Responses of Mexican Americans to Medical Treatment. Journal of Health and Social Behavior 8:299–308.

Neighbors, K.
    1969   Mexican American Folk Diseases. Western Folklore 28(4):249–259.

Padilla, A. M.
    1973   Latino Mental Health: Bibliography and Abstracts. U.S. Government Printing Office.

Pan American Health Organization
    1978   Selected Bibliography in Medical Anthropology for Health Professionals in the Americas. Field Office, Pan American Health Organization, El Paso, Texas.

Paredes, Americo
    1968   Folk Medicine and the Intercultural Jest. *In* Spanish-speaking People in the United States. June Helm, ed. pp. 104–119. Seattle: University of Washington Press.

Pattison, M.
    1973   Faith Healing: A Study of Personality and Function. Journal of Nervous and Mental Diseases 157:397–409.

Perez, Soledad
    1949   Mexican Folklore in Austin. M.A. thesis, University of Texas.

Press, Irwin
    1971   The Urban Curandero. American Anthropologist 73:741–756.

1978   Urban Folk Medicine. American Anthropologist 78(1): 71–84.

Quesada, Gustavo M., and Peter L. Heller
1977   Sociocultural Barriers to Medical Care among Mexican Americans in Texas. Medical Care 15(5):97–101.

Robbins, Russel Hope
1959   The Encyclopedia of Witchcraft and Demonology. New York: Crown.

Romano, Octavio
1960   Donship in a Mexican American Community in Texas. American Anthropologist 62:966–976.
1964   Don Pedrito Jaramillo: The Emergence of a Mexican American Folk Saint. Ph.D. dissertation, University of California, Berkeley.
1965   Charismatic Medicine, Folk-Healing, and Folk Sainthood. American Anthropologist 67:1151–1173.
1969   The Anthropology and Sociology of the Mexican-American History. El Grito, vol. 2.
1970   Social Science, Objectivity, and the Chicanos. El Grito, vol. 4.

Rubel, A. J.
1960   Concepts of Disease in a Mexican-American Community in Texas. American Anthropologist 62:795–814.
1964   The Epidemiology of a Folk Illness: Susto in Hispanic America. Ethnology 3:268–83.
1966   Across the Tracks: Mexican-Americans in a Texas City. Austin: University of Texas Press.
1969   El Susto en Hispanomerica. Revista de Ciencias Sociales, vol. 13.

Rubel, Arthur J., and Carl W. O'Nell
1978   Difficulties of Presenting Complaints to Physicians: Susto Illness an Example. In Modern Medicine and Medical Anthropology in the United States–Mexico Border Population. Boris Velimirovic, ed. Washington, D.C.: Pan American Health Organization. Scientific Publication no. 359.

Ruiz, P., and J. Langrod
1976a   Psychiatry and Folk Healing: A Dichotomy? American Journal of Psychiatry 133:95–97.
1976b   Role of Folk Healers in Community Mental Health Services. Community Mental Health Journal 12:392–398.

Samora, Julian
  1961   Conceptions of Disease among Spanish Americans. American Catholic Sociological Review 22:314–323.

Samora, Julian, et al.
  1961   Medical Vocabulary Knowledge among Hospital Patients. Journal of Health and Human Behavior 2:83–92.

Sanchez, Armand
  1971   The Definers and the Defined: A Mental Health Issue. El Grito, vol. 4

Saunders, Lyle
  1954   Cultural Differences and Medical Care: The Case of the Spanish-speaking People of the Southwest. New York: Russell Sage Foundation.
  1956   Cultural Factors Affecting Public Health Programs in a Border Agricultural Area. 14th Annual Meeting of the U.S.–Mexico Border Public Health Association. Calexico-Mexicali, 13–16 April.
  1958   Healing Ways in the Spanish Southwest. *In* Patients, Physicians and Illness. E. Gartley Jaco, ed. pp. 189–206. New York: Free Press.

Saunders, Lyle, and G. W. Hewes
  1953   Folk Medicine and Medical Practice. Journal of Medical Education 28:43–46.

Schendel, Gordon
  1968   Medicine in Mexico. Austin: University of Texas Press.

Schreiber, Janet M., and Loralee Philpott
  1978   Midwifery in the Lower Rio Grande Valley. *In* Modern Medicine and Medical Anthropology in the United States–Mexico Border Population. Boris Velimirovic, ed. Washington, D.C.: Pan American Health Organization. Scientific Publication no. 359.

Schulman, S., and A. M. Smith
  1953   The Concept of "Health" Among Spanish-speaking Villages in New Mexico and Colorado. Journal of Health and Human Behavior, pp. 226–234.

Scott, Florence Johnson
  1923   Customs and Superstitions among Texas Mexicans. Publications of the Texas Folklore Society 2:75–85.

Scrimshaw, Susan C. M., and Elizabeth Burleigh
  1978   The Potential for the Integration of Indigenous and West-

ern Medicines in Latin America and Hispanic Populations in the United States of America. *In* Modern Medicine and Medical Anthropology in the United States–Mexico Border Population. Boris Velimirovic, ed. Washington, D.C.: Pan American Health Organization. Scientific Publication no. 359.

Smithers, W. D.
1961   Nature's Pharmacy and the Curanderos. Alpine, Tex.: Sul Ross State College. Bulletin no. 51.

Snow, Loudell F.
1974   Folk Medical Beliefs and Their Implications for Care of Patients. Annals of Internal Medicine 81:82–96.

Speilberg, Joseph
1959   Social and Cultural Configurations and Medical Care: A Study of Mexican-Americans' Response to Proposed Hospitalization for the Treatment of Tuberculosis. M.A. thesis, University of Texas.

Timmreck, T. C.
1977   Folk Medicine and Healing among Spanish Speaking and Latin Americans. TPHA Journal (Jan.–Feb) pp. 77–90.

Torrey, E. Fuller
1969   The Case for the Indigenous Therapist. Archives of General Psychiatry 20(3):365–373.
1970   The Irrelevancy of Traditional Mental Health Services for Urban Mexican-Americans. Paper presented at the American Orthopsychiatry Association, San Francisco.
1972   The Mind Game: Witchdoctors and Psychiatrists. New York: Bantam Books.

Trotter, Robert T., II
1979   Evidence of an Ethnomedical Form of Aversion Therapy on the United States–Mexico Border. Journal of Ethnopharmacology 1(3):279–284.
1980   Remedios Caseros: Mexican American Home Remedies and Community Health Problems. Social Science and Medicine. In press.

Trotter, Robert T., II, and Juan Antonio Chavira
1978   Discovering New Models for Alcohol Counseling in Minority Groups. *In* Modern Medicine and Medical Anthropology in the United States–Mexico Border Population. Boris Velimirovic, ed. Washington, D.C.: Pan

American Health Organization. Scientific Publication no. 359.

Turner, Victor W.
   1969   The Ritual Process. Chicago: Aldine.

Unknown
   1951   Rudo Ensayo. By an unknown Jesuit. Tucson: Arizona Silhouettes Publication. 1st ed. 1763. Johann Nentuig, trans.

Uzzell, Douglas
   1974   Susto Revisited: Illness as a Strategic Role. American Ethnologist 1(2): 369–378.

Valvarde, Mark
   1972   Health Care of Urban Mexican Americans in a Southwestern City: A Preliminary Report of Findings. Galveston: University of Texas Medical Branch.

Velimirovic, Boris, ed.
   1978   Modern Medicine and Medical Anthropology in the United States–Mexico Border Population. Washington, D.C.: Pan American Health Organization. Scientific Publication no. 359.

Velimirovic, Boris, and Helga Velimirovic
   1978   The Utilization of Traditional Medicine and Its Practitioners in Health Services. In Modern Medicine and Medical Anthropology in the United States–Mexico Border Population. Boris Velimirovic, ed. Washington, D.C.: Pan American Health Organization. Scientific Publication no. 359.

Wagner, Federico
   n.d.   Remedios caseros con plantas medicinales. Mexico, D.F.: Medicina Hermanos.

Weclew, R. V.
   1975   The Nature, Prevalence and Levels of Awareness of "Curanderismo" and Some of Its Implications for Community Mental Health. Community Mental Health Journal 11: 145–154.

White, Beatrice Blyth
   1950   Paiute Sorcery. Viking Fund Publication in Anthropology no. 15. New York: Werner Gren Foundation.

Williams, Coleen
    1959 Cultural Differences and Medical Care of Ten Mexican
          Migrant Families in San Antonio, Texas. M.A. thesis,
          University of Texas.

Young, Allen
    1975 Some Implications of Medical Beliefs and Practices
          for Social Anthropology. American Anthropologist
          77:5–21.

INDEX